ROENTGENOLOGY OF
FRACTURES AND DISLOCATIONS

A Seminars in Roentgenology Reprint
January and April 1978

ROENTGENOLOGY OF FRACTURES AND DISLOCATIONS

Edited by

Benjamin Felson, M.D.

Professor, Department of Radiology
University of Cincinnati College of Medicine
Cincinnati, Ohio

GRUNE & STRATTON

A Subsidiary of Harcourt Brace Jovanovich, Publishers

New York   London   Toronto   Sydney   San Francisco

Library of Congress Cataloging in Publication Data

Main entry under title:

Roentgenology of fractures and dislocations.

  Bibliography: p.
  Includes index.
  1. Fractures—Diagnosis. 2. Dislocations—
Diagnosis. 3. Diagnosis, Radioscopic.
4. Radiography in orthopedia. I. Felson, Benjamin.
II. Seminars in roentgenology.
  RD102.R63   617'.15   78-15982
  ISBN 0-8089-1131-7

The chapters of this book originally appeared in the January and April 1978 issues (Volume XIII, Numbers 1 and 2) of *Seminars in Roentgenology,* a quarterly journal published by Grune and Stratton, Inc., and edited by Benjamin Felson, M.D.

Grune & Stratton, Inc.
111 Fifth Avenue
New York, New York 10003

Distributed in the United Kingdom by
Academic Press, Inc. (London) Ltd.
24/28 Oval Road, London NW 1

Library of Congress Catalog Number 78-15982
International Standard Book Number 0-8089-1131-7

Printed in the United States of America

CONTENTS

ROENTGENOLOGY OF
FRACTURES AND DISLOCATIONS

Letter From the Editor

"FRACTURES? In this era of CT scanning? Ridiculous!" You paid your subscription, so you're entitled to a reply as to why I selected such a prosaic topic, one that you already know so well, or think you do.

But first let me ask *you* some questions. When you see an unusual fracture, where do you go to look it up? Did your instructors teach you much about fractures during your residency? Did your department have a fracture conference? Did you attend? Have you or any of your medical acquaintances been sued for malpractice in a fracture case?

These nonrhetorical questions indicate the purpose of the next two Seminars. There have been many articles and a few books on the roentgenology of fractures, but a modern, concise, inclusive text devoted to the subject is not available. It is hoped that these Fracture Seminars will serve this purpose, encompassing newer concepts in the mechanisms, diagnosis, and treatment of fractures and re-expressing information your teachers knew but forgot to tell you.

Most training programs leave the resident to his own devices in the fracture area. When he brings a problem case to the attention of one of the staff members, he gets a quick yes or no and little discussion. There are, of course, gamesmanship cases shown at the radiology conference to trap the unwary: perilunate fracture, radial head dislocation, obscure fracture line, displaced fat pad, posterior dislocation of the humeral head. But a discussion of general principles applicable to future patients is seldom forthcoming.

The medicolegal actions related to bone trauma have reached epidemic proportions. This is now abating somewhat, probably as a result of countersuits instituted by defendant radiologists, claiming frivolous harrassment, better known as a *foul.* I have always accepted the widely expressed statement that many radiographs are taken on patients with trivial injuries purely for medicolegal protection.* I was shocked to discover recently that the percentage of such instances in emergency rooms is now claimed to be small (6.1%).**

From the patient's standpoint as well as for medicolegal reasons, the difference between "fracture" and "no fracture" is of considerable importance. To see a patient stretched out in skeletal traction via cranial burr holes for a nonexistent cervical spine dislocation is to be convinced. My young son once missed much of the baseball season because of a cast on his pitching arm. His injury occurred on the day that a famous radiologist, an expert on bone, was Visiting Professor in our department. The roentgenograms showed a line in the radius which the visitor and two of our own full professors agreed was a fracture. I had my doubts but, because of my obvious parental bias, I deferred to my more objective colleagues. Three weeks later the cast fell apart when the kid tried to pitch again. It was removed and a new film showed no callus and no fracture line. I eventually confessed the truth to the boy, but not until the statute of limitations had expired. (Can a son sue a father?) My son has since rejected radiology as an effective specialty.

Would you be embarrassed if a medical house officer puts up a chest film on your viewbox and points to a fresh rib fracture that you missed? It hurt my pride, though I realized he had the advantage of knowing that the patient had fallen out of bed and had point tenderness. The late Tom Hughes, the orderly who willed our Radiology Department $20,000 from his accumulated unspent wages, was our expert on rib fractures. He was so accurate that on all chest injuries we insisted Tommy look for and arrow the fractures that we otherwise might miss. One day I discovered his secret. Enroute to the x-ray department with a trauma victim, he stopped at a hallway recess and found out where the patient hurt. He was lousy with spine fractures, though: he did not understand referred pain.

Rib and transverse process fractures are in themselves not so important but they are a signpost pointing to the site of the injury and a warning that the trauma was reasonably severe. Armed with this information, the radiologist should know where to concentrate in his search for an accompanying visceral injury. Fracture of a lower left rib should make you consider rupture of the spleen, left kidney, or diaphragm, or

---

*Letter From Editor. Semin Roentgenol 9:87, 1974.

**Bulletin, American College of Radiology 33:1, Aug. 1977.

duodenal hematoma. Lumbar transverse process fracture raises the possibility of ruptured kidney or duodenum or injury to the pancreas. Fracture of the sternum should cause you to think of aortic laceration, bronchial tear, or cardiac injury.

It is surprising how often a pathologic fracture is assumed to be an ordinary traumatic fracture and its progressive destruction hidden under a thick cast. Conversely, a stress fracture or healing fracture may be mistaken for a benign or malignant tumor, both radiographically and histologically. Many fractures are set and casted by nonradiologists who are inexperienced in the radiologic recognition of local or systemic bone diseases. The radiologist who delegates his responsibility of fracture interpretation to the orthopedist is adding insult to the injury. Both specialists must interpret the films, together or apart.

We're all aware of the value of multiple views and the use of a grid and cone for demonstrating a fracture. But there are other technical tricks extremely useful to demonstrate or exclude a fracture or dislocation in problem cases. Tomography of the upper cervical spine is now widely employed. but have you used tomography to determine the status of a fracture within a cast? Image-amplified fluoroscopy with spot films is a great way to demonstrate a subtle

fracture. Years ago, we went to considerable effort to diagnose depressed skull fracture. We tried to gauge the plane of the fracture from the routine films and site of injury and obtain a tangential view of it. This was usually effective but often time-consuming. Now you can place the patient on the fluoroscopic table, turn his head until you see the fracture tangentially, and then spot-film it. The C-arm fluoroscope is even better for this purpose.

We've also found fluoroscopy useful in recognizing navicular, greenstick, cervical spine, and other fractures. It is a simple, quick, accurate way to be sure that there is or is not a fracture. It is amazing how well you can see a fracture line when you profile it with modern fluoroscopy, and how well you can show it with spot films.

So this is where we are: Fractures are among the most common conditions that the radiologist encounters, and a frequent source of litigation. Yet we deal with them casually, often relegating them to the novice. The least we can do is teach him and provide him with an adequate reference book. And maybe it wouldn't hurt to read it ourselves.

Benjamin Felson, M.D.
Editor

Normal Skull Variants That May Simulate a Fracture

Thomas A. Tomsick

1. Artifact or soft tissue alteration (eg, skin laceration, skin fold, air trapped beneath skin, matted hair, hair braid, rubber band, tape, dressing, linen
2. Arterial groove[1,3] (eg, meningeal vessels, middle temporal branch of superficial temporal artery, deep temporal branches of internal maxillary artery, supraorbital artery)
3. Emissary vein, venous lake, diploic channel, sinus groove[1,3]
4. Fissure, synchondrosis, suture, sutural (Wormian) bone
   a. Cerebellar synchondrosis[2,3]
   b. Coronal suture[6]
   c. Innominate synchondrosis[6]
   d. Intersphenoid synchondrosis[3]
   e. Intraparietal suture[4]
   f. Lambdoid suture[6]
   g. Lateral fissures of the foramen magnum[1,2]
   h. Lateral interparietal fissure[1]
   i. Lateral sphenoidal sutures[1]
   j. Median occipital fissures[1,2]
   k. Mendosal suture[6]
   l. Metopic suture[1,3]
   m. Occipitomastoid suture[6]
   n. Parietal fissure[1,6]
   o. Parietomastoid suture[6]
   p. Spheno-occipital synchondrosis[6]
   q. Squamosal suture[1,6]
   r. Transverse occipital suture[1]
   s. Unfused planum sphenoidale[5]

REFERENCES

1. Allen WE, Kier EL, Rothman SLG: Pitfalls in the evaluation of skull trauma. Radiol Clin North Am 11:479–503, 1973

2. Franken EA: The midline occipital fissure: Diagnosis of fracture versus anatomic variant. Radiology 93:1043–1046, 1969

3. Keats TE: Roentgen Variants That May Simulate Disease. Chicago, Illinois, Yearbook Medical Publishers, 1973, pp 3–65

4. Shapiro R: Anomalous parietal sutures and the bipartite parietal bone. Am J Roentgenol 115:569–577, 1972

5. Smith TR, Kier EL: The unfused planum sphenoidale: Differentiation from fracture. Radiology 98:305–309, 1971

6. Swischuk LE: The normal pediatric skull: Variations and artefacts. Radiol Clin North Am 10:277–290, 1972

Thomas A. Tomsick, M.D.: *Assistant Professor of Radiology, University of Cincinnati College of Medicine, Department of Radiology, Cincinnati General Hospital, Cincinnati, Ohio.*

© 1978 by Grune & Stratton, Inc.
0037-198X/78/1301-0008 $1.00/0

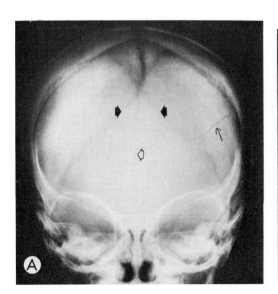 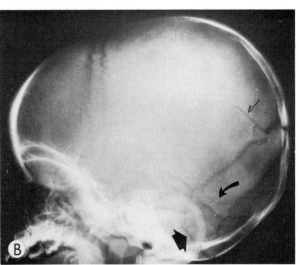

Fig. 1.   This girl had a frontal head injury. Note the intraparietal suture (thin black arrows), metopic suture (open arrow), interparietal or Inca bone (small closed arrows), mendosal suture (curved arrow), and innominate synchondrosis (large arrow).

Pseudofractures and Stress Fractures

Ronald Grusd

Pseudofractures

Common

1. Osteomalacia
2. Paget disease
3. Rickets
4. [Spondylolysis]*
5. [Stress fractures]

Uncommon

1. Diaphyseal aclasia
2. Fibrous dysplasia (including Albright syndrome)
3. Hyperphosphatasia
4. Hypophosphatasia
5. Surgery (eg, graft donor site)
6. Neuropathic disorders (eg, leprosy)
7. Osteogenesis imperfecta
8. Osteopetrosis, pyknodysostosis
9. Osteoporosis
10. Radiation osteitis
11. Renal osteodystrophy
12. Rheumatoid arthritis
13. Steroid therapy, Cushing syndrome

SUBGAMUT

Stress Fractures

1. Athlete: midtibia (shinsplints), pubis
2. Ballet dancer: midtibia
3. Chronic coughing: lower ribs; dyspnea: first rib
4. Clay-shoveler: cervicodorsal spinous process
5. Golfer: ribs
6. Heavy-pack-bearer: first rib
7. Long-distance runner: distal fibula, midtibia
8. March fracture: metatarsal, other bones
9. Parachutist: proximal fibula
10. Pitchfork-handler: ulna
11. Standing: calcaneus, metatarsal sesamoid
12. Stooping: obturator ring
13. Tic: clavicle
14. Trapshooter: coracoid

*Brackets indicate entities that can be confused with pseudofractures.

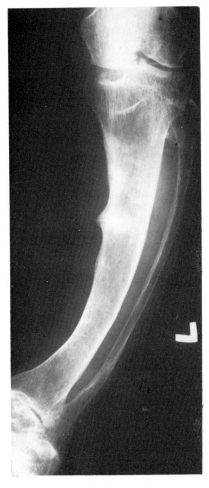

Fig. 1. Osteomalacia of unknown etiology with pseudofractures.

REFERENCES

1. Greenfield GB: Radiology of Bone Diseases (ed 2). Philadelphia, JB Lippincott, 1975
2. Murray RO, Jacobson HG: The Radiology of Skeletal

Ronald Grusd, M.D.: *Assistant Professor of Radiology, University of Cincinnati College of Medicine; Department of Radiology, Cincinnati General Hospital, Cincinnati, Ohio.*

Reprint requests should be addressed to Dr. Ronald Grusd, Department of Radiology, Cincinnati General Hospital, Cincinnati, Ohio 45267.
© 1978 by Grune & Stratton, Inc.
0037-198X/78/1302-0001$0100/0

Disorders vols 1–3 (ed 2). New York, Churchill Livingstone, 1977

3. Rasad S: Golfer's fractures of the ribs. Report of 3 cases. Am J Roentgenol 120:901–903, 1974

4. Reeder MM, Felson B: Gamuts in Radiology. Cincinnati, Audiovisual Radiology of Cincinnati, 1975, D-72

5. Sandrock A: Radiographic exhibit. Stress fracture of the coracoid process of the scapula. Radiology 117:274, 1975

6. Schneider R, Kaye JJ: Insufficiency and stress fractures of the long bones occurring in patients with rheumatoid arthritis. Radiology 116:595–599, 1975

The Radiologist, the Orthopedist, the Lawyer, and the Fracture

Robert R. Renner, George G. Mauler, and J. Lee Ambrose

THIS ARTICLE will explore the common radiologic problem of bone trauma and the relationship between the orthopedic surgeon and the radiologist. Skeletal trauma represents 34% of the radiologic practice at Cortland Memorial Hospital, a 175-bed hospital serving a population of 50,000. Included within the service area are two ski resorts, a large state university physical education program, and an interstate highway.

THE PROBLEM

We believe that a problem exists in regard to the interaction between the radiologist and the orthopedic surgeon. Typically, the problem may be illustrated in a university hospital, in which the considerable separation between the departments of orthopedic surgery and radiology results in the patient waiting in the radiology department for his films to be taken and read while the orthopedic surgeon becomes angry at the delay in his return. The chief of orthopedic surgery may then talk the hospital administrators into placing a radiographic unit in the orthopedic department. Another facet of the problem concerns the radiographic unit in the emergency room. Films made of a possible fracture may be viewed and acted on by the orthopedic surgeon and only subsequently interpreted by the radiology resident. Even if the radiology resident reads the films first, he is seldom supervised by a radiologist experienced in bone trauma, and his report is generally ignored. Follow-up films on the fracture are often reported by the radiology resident without knowledge of the therapy employed, the orthopedist's problems, or the acceptable limits of displacement. When the orthopedist comes to the radiology department to view fracture films, he is usually accompanied by his house staff, and he asks for radiologic assistance only when a question of pathologic fracture arises. The radiology resident often develops an interest in rare bone pathology, but he looks on the common fracture as a routine dictation chore.

The problem, unfortunately, spills over into the community hospital, where Figure 1 depicts a common scene. Radiologic reports on bone trauma continue to be poor and sometimes ridiculous. They are often late in arriving on the chart and are frequently ignored. Often a significant fracture will be dismissed by the radiologist as "an orthopedic problem" and quickly and routinely dictated. A mutual lack of professional respect develops.

The legal profession is also involved in the problem. Although the growth rate of malpractice suits is declining, each year more suits occur and higher judgments are awarded. The orthopedic surgeon continues to have a high exposure risk, since most of the suits involve fracture diagnosis or treatment. Also, malpractice lawyers have discovered that radiologists can be sued for missed diagnoses or delayed reports.

Formerly, hospitals were legally liable only if their custodial care of patients was negligent. There was no liability for negligent acts of a physician unless the physician was employed by the hospital. Now, since federal and state laws require utilization review and medical audit, the public is increasingly looking to the hospital as an institutional provider of medical care. A legal doctrine is developing that the hospital must control the quality of medical care provided by its organized medical staff and that it is liable for failure to do so.[13] This hospital liability has been extended to physician conduct in those situations where the hospital controls the contractual relationship and there is no free choice of physician, as in radiology.[2] Recent

Robert R. Renner, M.D., J.D.: *Associate Clinical Professor of Radiology, Upstate Medical Center, Syracuse, N.Y.; Department of Radiology, Cortland Memorial Hospital, Cortland, N.Y. (Dr. Renner is also an attorney.)* George G. Mauler, M.D.: *Clinical Instructor, Department of Orthopedic Surgery, Upstate Medical Center, Syracuse, N.Y.; Department of Orthopedic Surgery, Cortland Memorial Hospital, Cortland, N.Y.* J. Lee Ambrose, M.D.: *Assistant Clinical Professor, Department of Radiology, Upstate Medical Center, Syracuse, N.Y.; Department of Radiology, Cortland Memorial Hospital, Cortland, N.Y.*

Reprint requests should be addressed to Dr. Robert R. Renner, Department of Radiology, Cortland Memorial Hospital, Cortland, N.Y. 13045.

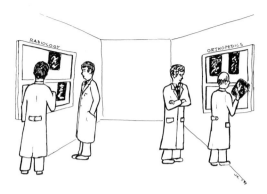

Fig. 1.   Radiologists and orthopedic surgeons study their films separately.

court decisions have also implied that the hospital's liability can extend to acts of private practitioners when its medical staff bylaws have been violated or its committees have failed to function properly.[3,4,9,14] Like physician malpractice insurance, hospital malpractice insurance has become more difficult to obtain and considerably more expensive. Soon all hospitals will likely have programs of risk management. A key factor in such programs will be the interaction between medical specialists, with particular attention being paid to the radiology department's interaction with other components of the hospital.

Just as much radiology in this country is still done by nonradiologists, much bone trauma is managed by nonorthopedists. In either case, the handling of bone trauma may be of poor quality. The nonorthopedist often seeks the advice of the radiologist, who, if he understands bone trauma and its management, is in a good position to direct adequate care and secure orthopedic referral when it is necessary.

We believe that the problem should be attacked squarely by radiologists who recognize it in their institutions. Besides such simple personal amenities as improving communication and showing concern for the patient, the radiologist should do the following:

1. Learn and use basic orthopedic terminology.
2. Give "same hour" or "next morning" reports, and make them concise.
3. Call the orthopedic surgeon when unsure or when concerned.
4. Maintain excellent technical quality for all films.
5. Take enough views to show the pathology.

6. Mark films clearly, and show elapsed time from initial injury.
7. Maintain a ready reference library on bone trauma.
8. Develop an interest in the subject of fractures.

BIOMECHANICAL PRINCIPLES

First, let us consider elementary biomechanical principles. A fracture is a failure of bone as a material and as a structure. As a material, bone is much stronger in compression than in tension, and many fractures are failure of bone under tension loading. The response of a small piece of wet bone in tension loading can be shown on a stress–strain graph (Fig. 2). Stress is the force per unit area that develops on a certain plane when force is applied. Strain is the percentage deformation that occurs. Note that these figures are "normalized" by unit area and percentage change so that they are characteristic of bony material in general.

As bone is first loaded, there is a linear relationship between deformation and stress. In this situation, as the bone is then unloaded, it returns to its original shape, and is said to be elastic. With loading beyond the yield point, bone retains some deformation when it is unloaded; this property is termed plastic. The sudden vertical termination in Figure 2 is the failure or fracture point. Since work = force × distance, the area under the curve represents work put into the bone (the actual energy stored in the bone at any level of loading). Bone is much stronger in compression; it does not fail dramatically, but rather in a slow, cruising fashion (Fig. 3).

Other factors affect bone failure, notably the rapidity of loading and the associated energy-

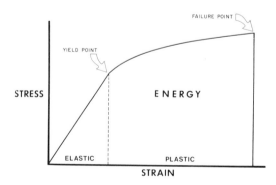

Fig. 2.   Response of wet bone in tension loading.

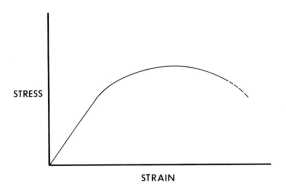

Fig. 3. Response of wet bone in compression loading.

absorbing systems, especially the muscles. If bone is loaded rapidly, it will tolerate greater deformation and absorb more energy; but if it then fractures, this greater level of stored energy will produce far greater bone damage and comminution. Muscles dissipate much of the force directed to bone, and many fractures are the result of muscular or neuromuscular disturbance of this protective mechanism.[5]

The likelihood of failure (or fracture) is also greatly influenced by the architectural structure of bone. For example, a bone with a single screw hole has only one-half its former loading tolerance and only one-fourth its former energy-storing capacity. Loss of secondary "strut" trabeculae in osteoporosis results in considerable weakness, despite hypertrophy of the primary trabeculae.

TERMINOLOGY

Types of Fractures (Fig. 4)

Open Fracture

An open fracture is one in which there is communication between the fracture and the outside environment. *Compound fracture* has been a confusing term. An open fracture is a surgical emergency. Any fracture with an adjacent wound is assumed to be an open fracture until proved otherwise.

Closed Fracture

A closed fracture is one that does not communicate with the outside environment.

Incomplete Fracture

An incomplete fracture is a stable fracture with a broken cortex but in which the bone is not in complete discontinuity; for example, the following children's fractures:

Greenstick fracture. With angular stress, the cortex opens on the convex side.

Torus fracture. With angular stress, the cortex buckles or folds like an accordion on the concave side.

Avulsion Fracture

An avulsion fracture involves a pulling loose of a bony insertion by a muscle or ligament.

Impaction Fracture

In an impaction fracture a fragment of bone is driven or telescoped into the opposing fragment. Some specific impaction fractures are the following:

Depression fracture. A hard surface of bone is driven into soft adjacent bone, as in tibial plateau depression.

Compression fracture. Compression fracture characteristically occurs in the spine. With forceful flexion, the vertebral endplates are forced toward each other, compressing the intervening spongy bone.

Comminuted Fracture

A comminuted fracture is one with more than two fragments. This also includes special subcategories:

Butterfly fragment. A butterfly fragment is a wedge-shaped third fragment of a long bone fracture at the apex of the force input.

Segmental fracture. Two fracture lines isolate a discrete segment of the shaft of a long bone.

Pathologic Fracture

A pathologic fracture is fracture through bone weakened by a disease process.

Fatigue Fracture

A fatigue fracture involves discontinuity of a bone caused by repetitive stress, with gradual interruption in its structure at a greater rate than can be offset by the reparative process. The term *stress fracture* is frequently used, but *fatigue fracture* more precisely describes the mechanism peculiar to this injury.

Configurations of Fractures (Fig. 5)

The configuration of a fracture often represents a visible image of the force of the

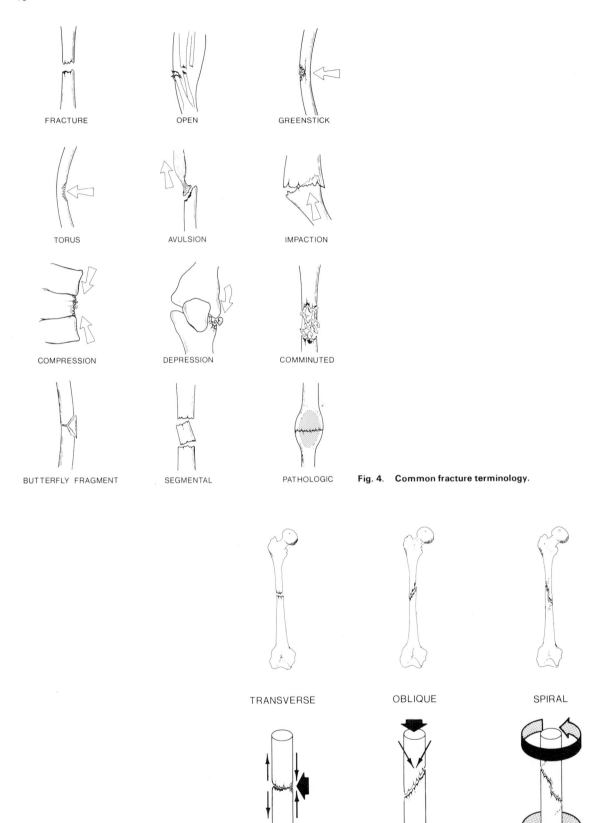

FRACTURE   OPEN   GREENSTICK

TORUS   AVULSION   IMPACTION

COMPRESSION   DEPRESSION   COMMINUTED

BUTTERFLY FRAGMENT   SEGMENTAL   PATHOLOGIC

Fig. 4.   Common fracture terminology.

TRANSVERSE   OBLIQUE   SPIRAL

Fig. 5.   Configurations and mechanisms of common long bone fractures.

fracture mechanism. The three most common fracture configurations are the following:

Transverse

With angular stress, the bone undergoes deformation. The collagen fibers on the convex side undergo tensile failure, and the mineral structure on the concave side undergoes failure in compression.

Oblique

The oblique configuration occurs with axial loading, when there is a resolution of forces at 45 degrees to the axis. The fracture occurs along the path of least resistance.

Spiral

In spiral fracture, material failure of bone occurs because of rotatory stress. Note that there is a short, straight vertical portion that is the initial area of bone failure; the spiral legs then propagate in each direction.

Location of Fracture

The long bone is conveniently divided into thirds for description of the fracture site. For example: the fracture lies at the junction of the proximal third and the middle third of the tibia; the fracture lies within the middle third and the distal third of the radius. These may be abbreviated PM 3 and DM 3). Intra-articular extension of the fracture is always mentioned. Many other special terms are used with individual fractures, but they are less standardized.

Position of Fracture Fragments (Fig. 6)

Alignment

The angulation of a fracture is described as the position of the distal fragment in relation to the proximal fragment. If there is no perceptible angulation, the fracture is said to be in good alignment. Descriptive terms such as internal and external and radial and ulnar are self-explanatory. Varus and valgus are often described in relation to alignment. Varus is a bending inward of a distal fragment toward the midline of the body. Valgus is a bending outward of a distal fragment away from the midline of the body.

Apposition

Apposition concerns the state of bony contact at the fracture site. A fracture with complete surface area contact is said to be in complete or good apposition. When there is partial contact, it is said to be in partial apposition. When the fracture ends overlap, it is described as being in overlapping or bayonet apposition. If the fracture ends are pulled apart by muscle force or therapeutic traction, it is said to be in distraction.

Rotation

Twisting displacement of a fractured bone about its longitudinal axis is called rotation. Frequently roentgenograms are not as valuable as clinical examination in determining rotational displacement. The radiologist must be careful not to conclude or imply too much from the roentgenographic appearance. In many instances it might be better to state that the fracture is "in excellent alignment and apposition" rather than "in excellent position," because the latter implies an adequacy of rotational reduction that often cannot be perceived on a roentgenogram. Inclusion of the proximal and distal joints on the film is helpful in determining rotation.

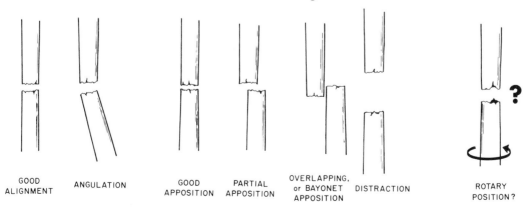

GOOD ALIGNMENT ANGULATION GOOD APPOSITION PARTIAL APPOSITION OVERLAPPING, or BAYONET APPOSITION DISTRACTION ROTARY POSITION?

Fig. 6.   Position terminology for long bone fractures.

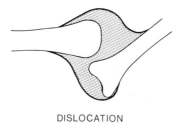

DISLOCATION

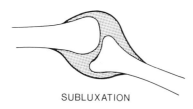

SUBLUXATION

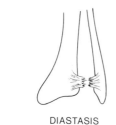

DIASTASIS

Fig. 7. Common joint derangements.

Joint Derangements (Fig. 7)

Dislocation

Dislocation means complete loss of contact between the usual articular surface components of a joint.

Subluxation

Subluxation means partial loss of contact between the usual articular surface components of a joint.

Diastasis

Diastasis means frank separation of a slightly movable joint, most often the pubic symphysis or the distal tibiofibular syndesmosis.

Fracture Healing

Bone must be considered as a dynamic and living tissue. Its blood supply is all-important; no osteocyte resides more than 10 μ away from its arterial supply. There are three basic types of fracture healing:

Endochondral

Endochondral healing is the classic cortical healing in tubular long bone fractures. It is similar to epiphyseal plate growth activity, but less ordered. Endochondral fracture healing is subdivided into three main phases that overlap chronologically:

Inflammatory phase. The fracture (Fig. 8) occurs in a soft-tissue envelope containing torn periosteum, muscles, and numerous blood vessels. The resulting hematoma becomes clotted. The bone ends in the immediate vicinity die because their periosteal blood supply is stripped. This is further enhanced with surgical stripping of the periosteum. Necrotic material causes an inflammatory response. Osteoblast proliferation occurs over the entire bone within 18 hours. Hyperemia of the entire bone develops.

Reparative phase. The hematoma (Fig. 9) then undergoes organization. Recent work has indicated that the hematoma does not contribute cells to bone healing and that, if anything, it acts as an inhibiting mechanical block to healing. Stem cells from the periosteum, endosteum, and haversian canal lining form osteoblasts and chondroblasts. Along with the increased blood supply to the entire limb, there is an ingrowth of capillary buds, mainly from the periosteal vessels. The chondroid and osteoid gradually envelop the bone ends, increasing the stability of the fracture. Low oxygen tension favors cartilage formation; higher oxygen tension favors bone formation. Therefore cartilage predominates in early healing and primary bone in later healing. Bone mineral, calcium hydroxyapatite, is deposited initially in spaces in the collagen lattice of the ground substance called "hole zones." The final volume distribution of mineral lies in these hole zones. This initial loosely woven bone, which is not oriented in response to stress, is called primary callus.

Remodeling phase. In 1892 Wolff stated that the architecture of a skeletal system corresponds to the mechanical needs of that system. In other words, form follows function. New strips of bone are laid down corresponding to the lines of force placed on the bone (Fig. 10). Poorly placed trabeculae are resorbed. Primary callus is slowly removed and replaced with new bone that follows the stress function of that

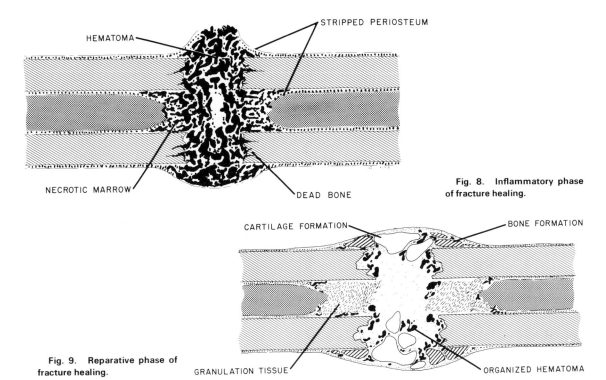

Fig. 8. Inflammatory phase of fracture healing.

Fig. 9. Reparative phase of fracture healing.

bone. It has recently been demonstrated that with stress deformation, electropositivity occurs on the convex surface and electronegativity on the concave surface by means of a piezoelectric effect.[1,6] Interestingly, electropositivity is associated with osteoblastic activity, causing the convex surface to smooth into a more linear configuration. Conversely, electronegativity is associated with osteoblastic activity, causing a filling of the concave surface. A fracture site becomes electronegative immediately and remains so until remodeling is complete. The electron may be the "first messenger" in the total sequence of physical-chemical function in

the bone system. Low-voltage direct current is now occasionally being used to promote bone healing in difficult fracture cases.[8]

Membranous

Membranous healing occurs in fractures with good fixation and contact, with or without compression. The fracture gap is filled with periosteal and endosteal new bone formation.

Primary

The primary or Swiss type of fracture healing occurs only in the experimental laboratory when a bone defect is made after a compression

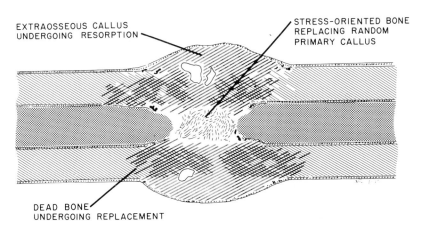

Fig. 10. Remodeling phase of fracture healing.

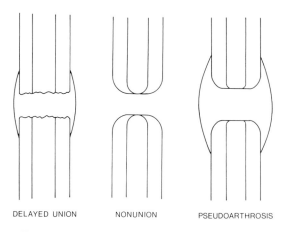

DELAYED UNION   NONUNION   PSEUDOARTHROSIS

Fig. 11. Delayed union and nonunion. Bone healing is usually progressing at the site of delayed union, but at a retarded rate. There is complete absence of bone healing in nonunion. The connective tissue at the site of a pseudarthrosis has formed a new joint space with a synovial lining.

plate is applied and compression is exerted. Supposedly this causes haversian canals formerly in continuity to reunite. Clinically, compression plating of a fracture results in membranous bone formation.

Abnormalities of Fracture Healing (Fig. 11)

Delayed Union

Delayed union is a failure to unite within the expected time, taking into consideration the patient, the bone involved, and the type of fracture. It is a matter of *clinical* appraisal. It may be due to local or systemic factors. Eventually the fracture usually proceeds to union.

Nonunion

Nonunion is cessation of bone healing. It is a matter of *radiographic* diagnosis. The ends of the fracture fragments become rounded and sclerotic. Medullary access to the fracture site is obliterated. The fracture site persists with little or no evidence of bony callus. The bony ends are usually joined by fibrous or fibrocartilaginous callus, but occasionally a false joint occurs and develops its own synovial lining. This is called a pseudarthrosis.

Malunion

Malunion is union of a fracture in an unacceptable position.

Aseptic Necrosis

Aseptic necrosis is bone death caused by interrupted blood supply. It was first described by Axhausen and was made more widely known by Phemister.[10] The dead bone is replaced by "creeping substitution." Often the bone becomes plastic and is easily deformed until it is fully remodeled.

FRACTURES IN CHILDREN

Children are not just small adults. The structures and functions of the child's skeletal system differ greatly from those of the adult.[11] Structurally, the child's bone has radiolucent growth cartilage that is not amenable to radiographic detection of injury. The periosteum of the child's bone is thicker and produces callus more rapidly and more abundantly than that of the adult. Biomechanically, the child's bone fails more slowly, because it has a more gradual and more prolonged phase of plastic deformation before eventual failure. Certain physiologic differences are very important in pediatric trauma:

Remodeling

With certain displaced fractures, remodeling can improve the result. Remodeling will generally help when the child has 2 years or more of growth ahead of him, when the fracture lies near the end of a long bone, or when angular deformity is in the plane of movement of the adjacent joint. Remodeling generally will not help if there are displaced intra-articular fractures, if the fracture is near the midshaft area of a long bone, if angular deformity is at a right angle to the plane of movement of the adjacent joint, or if a displaced fracture crosses the epiphyseal plate at a right angle.

Longitudinal Overgrowth

Longitudinal overgrowth occurs in many long bone fractures in children. The process of fracture healing includes hyperemia of the entire bone, which causes increased nutrition to the growth cartilage and thereby increases longitudinal growth. An undisplaced femoral fracture, on the average, will have about 1 cm overgrowth in about 1 year. This usually is not of great clinical significance. Many authorities believe that this is partially compensated for by premature closure of the epiphyses on the injured side.

Other Special Features

Progressive deformity can occur in children. Damage to the substance of an epiphyseal plate may produce shortening or a progressive angular deformity. Comminution is rare in children because the flexibility of a child's bone dissipates much of the force of impact. Nonunion is rare in children, and fractures generally heal rapidly.

Epiphyseal fractures comprise one-third of bone injuries in children. Understanding the anatomy of the epiphyseal area is crucial with these fractures (Fig. 12). The growth plate is a cartilaginous disk between the epiphysis and the metaphysis. Germinal cells are attached to the epiphysis; they get their blood supply from epiphyseal vessels. Multiplication of germinal cells increases the cell population of the plate. Daughter cells multiply further, secrete matrix, increase the size of the cartilage mass, and thereby cause growth. The matrix then calcifies. Metaphyseal vessels then enter cell columns, remove some of the matrix, and deposit bone on the cartilage to form the metaphysis.

Epiphyseal separation invariably occurs at the junction of the calcified matrix and the uncalcified matrix, where there is the least structural resistance to shearing stress. The important germinal layer and most of the thickness of the epiphyseal plate remain with the epiphysis. Most of the plane of the epiphyseal separation is bloodless; consequently there is little swelling associated with the injury.

Anyone involved in radiologic diagnosis of children's trauma should understand and use the Salter-Harris classification of epiphyseal injuries (Fig. 13).[12]

SALTER-HARRIS CLASSIFICATION

Type I fracture is a simple separation of the epiphysis. Germinal cells migrate with epiphysis, and the calcified matrix migrates with the metaphysis. If the periosteum is not torn, there is no displacement. The radiograph may be normal, the diagnosis being made clinically because of tenderness over the epiphyseal plate. Some orthopedists obtain stress films, but many prefer not to do so. Separation of an unossified epiphysis must be diagnosed early by clinical signs and soft-tissue swelling. Pathologic type I

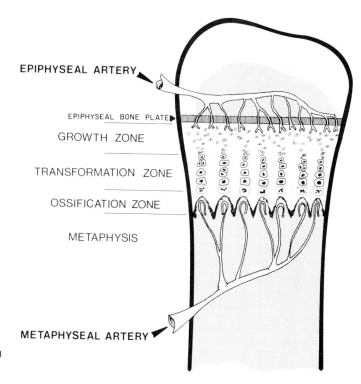

EPIPHYSEAL ARTERY

EPIPHYSEAL BONE PLATE

GROWTH ZONE

TRANSFORMATION ZONE

OSSIFICATION ZONE

METAPHYSIS

METAPHYSEAL ARTERY

Fig. 12. Anatomy of the epiphyseal area.

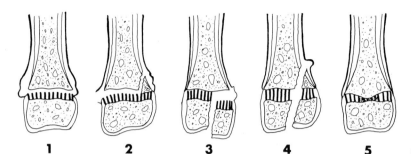

1   2   3   4   5

Fig. 13. Salter-Harris classification of epiphyseal injuries.

injuries occur in scurvy, rickets, osteomyelitis, and hormone imbalance.

In type II fracture, the plane of injury travels through most of the epiphysis and then a portion of the metaphysis. The metaphyseal fragment is called the Thurstan-Holland sign.[7] The epiphyseal separation is usually easily reduced.

Type III fracture is rare. The fracture passes through the growth plate and then the epiphysis. It is an intra-articular fracture, and it requires open reduction. The most common example is the Tillaux fracture of the tibia, which is actually an avulsion from the pull of the anterior tibiofibular ligament.

Type IV fracture passes through the joint surface, epiphysis, epiphyseal plate, and metaphysis. The most common location for this fracture is the lateral condyle of the humerus. Open reduction and internal fixation are usually necessary. Without good reduction, significant deformity is likely.

Type V fracture is a crushing of the epiphyseal plate, which causes growth arrest. Fortunately it is rare. Total epiphyseal arrest creates shortening, whereas partial arrest leads to progressive angular deformity. Initially the injury may be thought to be a sprain, since the radiographs are normal. A history of a large precipitating force, such as a fall from a significant height with longitudinal force loading, may be significant. Some type I or type II injuries may result in growth arrest. This is probably because they contain a component of type V injury. It is best to warn anyone with an epiphyseal injury that problems of this sort may occur. Every epiphyseal injury should be followed at least 1 year to ensure that the plate is normal, that there is no metaphyseal sclerosis, and that new bone develops beyond Harris' line, the scar of the injury.

THE WEAK-LINK CONCEPT

The nature and displacement of fractures are dependent on the magnitude and direction of the force, the pull of the affected muscles, and the so-called weak link. A direct blow may fracture the clavicle at the site of force, but the usual force resulting in fracture of the clavicle is lateral and is transmitted through the shoulder. It is because of the S shape of the clavicle that the fracture occurs at midshaft.

The displacing effect of muscle pull is well demonstrated in fractures of the humerus (Fig. 14). If the fracture is above the pectoralis major, the distal fracture fragment is pulled medially, while the proximal fragment is mildly abducted. A fracture below the level of the pectoralis major causes the proximal fracture fragment to be pulled medially, while the distal fragment is abducted by the deltoid pull. A fracture below the level of the deltoid results in abduction of the proximal fracture fragment and proximal displacement of the distal fragment by the pull of the coracobrachial muscle.

The weak-link concept varies with the patient's age. In the child, the junction between the zone of provisional calcification and the noncalcified chondroid in the epiphyseal plate constitutes the weak link. In the young athlete, whose epiphyseal plates are closed and whose bone is strong, the weak link is usually the ligamentous structure. In the elderly patient with osteoporotic bone, the weak link is commonly the bony trabeculae. For example, the injury caused by a valgus force applied to the knee joint will vary with the patient's age. In the youngster, the weak point is the epiphyseal plate. However, once the epiphyseal plate has closed and the bone is strong, the ligament becomes the weak point, and the same valgus

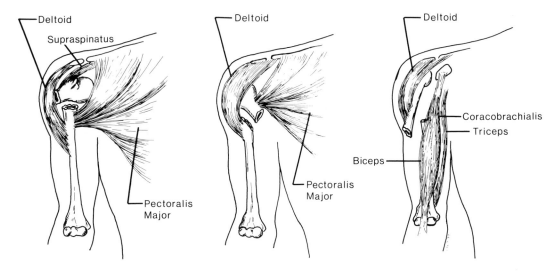

Fig. 14.   Effects of muscle pull on placement of fracture of the humerus at various levels.

stress force will rupture the ligament. As the patient grows older, bone strength decreases due to osteoporosis; in that case, the same valgus force will cause depression fractures of the tibial plateau. Another example is the upper extremity. A valgus force may avulse the medial epicondyle in a young adolescent, whereas in an adult the same force will fracture the softer radial head or neck (Fig. 15).

RESOLUTION OF THE PROBLEM

There is a great need for the radiologist to give early, concise reports and to communicate these reports to the orthopedic surgeon while the patient is waiting. A telephone call to discuss the case with the referring physician when the radiologist is unsure or is concerned about the abnormality will also be appreciated. If the orthopedic surgeon trusts the radiologist's interpretation, he can often begin the patient's treatment based on the telephoned report. This can save considerable time for the orthopedic surgeon. The radiologist and the orthopedic surgeon may each miss points on the films that the other finds. A close working relationship between them can result in earlier correct treatment of the patient.

Familiarity with the principles of bone and

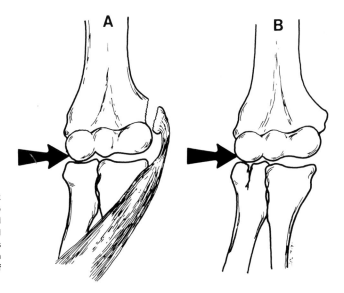

Fig. 15.   An example of the weak-link concept. (A) A valgus stress directed to the elbow in an adolescent has caused avulsion of the epiphysis of the medial humeral epicondyle. (B) The same valgus stress directed to the adult elbow often causes a chisel or depression fracture of the radial head.

ligament trauma will also lead to the taking of appropriate additional views to show the full extent of the injury; for example: ruling out a fracture at the base of the fifth metatarsal when an ankle fracture is suspected; obtaining a more proximal film when there is separation of the tibiofibular syndesmosis in order to show an associated fracture through the upper fibula.

We mark all our fracture films clearly with a black wax marking pencil. The initial films are marked "injury," and the time following injury is noted in days, weeks, months, or years. In addition, we usually write the date of the filming in bold numbers on the film. If there has been surgery, we may mark the films with sequential Roman numerals for the postoperative studies. Occasionally we indicate on portable films the position of the extremity, if this is not readily apparent. The marks not only enable the orthopedic surgeon to review the films quickly but also provide a significant teaching device in terms of timing of bone healing and maintenance of position. A final point: we make an effort to keep the films in sequential order in the front of the patient's film jacket.

The following is a list of orthopedic-oriented books that we recommend be kept at hand near the fracture reading area:

1. Basic fracture definitions and nomenclature: Schultz RJ: The Language of Fractures. Baltimore, Williams & Wilkins, 1972
2. Comprehensive fracture text: Rockwood CA, Green DP: Fractures. Philadelphia, Lippincott, 1975
3. Excellent and readable insights into children's fractures: Rang M: Children's Fractures. Philadelphia, Lippincott, 1974
4. Interesting collection of original descriptions and eponymic derivations in orthopedics and trauma: Rang M: Anthology of Orthopaedics. London, E&S Livingstone, 1966

Bone trauma can be an interesting subject, and its interest is automatically enhanced by a better understanding of the problems facing the othopedic surgeon. If the radiologist takes time to review the films with the orthopedic surgeon, they will gain knowledge beneficial to the patient and to each other.

ACKNOWLEDGMENTS

The authors thank Mrs. Joanne Rienhardt for her editorial assistance and Jim Rienhardt for the illustrations.

REFERENCES

1. Bassett CAL, Becker RO: Generation of electrical potentials by bone in response to mechanical stress. Science 137:1063–1064, 1962

2. Beeck v. Tucson General Hospital, 18 Ariz.App. 165, 500 P.2d 1153 (Ct. App. 1972)

3. Corleto v. Shore Memorial Hospital, 138 N.J.Sup. 302, 350 A.2d 534 (1975)

4. Darling v. Charleston Community Hospital, 33 Ill.2d 326, 211 N.E.2d 253 (1965), cert. denied 383 U.S. 946 (1966)

5. Frankel VH, Burstein AH: Orthopaedic Biomechanics: The Application of Engineering to the Musculoskeletal System. Philadelphia, Lea & Febiger, 1970

6. Fukada E, Yasuda I: On the piezoelectric effect of bone. J Physiol Soc Jpn 12:1158–1162, 1957

7. Holland CT: Radiographical note on injuries to distal epiphyses of radius and ulna. Proc R Soc Med 22:23–28, 1929

8. Lavine LS, Lustrin I, Shamos MH, Rinaldi RA, Liboff AR: Electrical enhancement of bone healing. Science 175:1118–1121, 1972 (abstract)

9. Pederson v. Dumouchel, 431 P.2d 973 (1967)

10. Phemister DB: Bone growth and repair (Arthur Dean Bevin lecture). Ann Surg 102:261–285, 1935

11. Rang M: Children's Fractures. Philadelphia, Lippincott, 1974

12. Salter RB, Harris WR: Injuries involving the epiphyseal plate. J Bone Joint Surg [Am] 45A:587–622, 1963

13. Southwick AF: The hospital as an institution—expanding responsibilities change its relationship with the staff physician. Calif West Law Rev 9:429–467, 1973

14. Tucson Medical Center, Incorporated v. Misevch, 113 Ariz. 34, 545 P.2d 958 (1976)

An Atlas of Simulated Fractures

Theodore E. Keats

The diagnostician must be familiar with normal variation if he is not to give his patients diseases which they do not have.

John Caffey

THE ABILITY to differentiate a true fracture from a simulated fracture is often what distinguishes the professional radiologist from the amateur. This ability is a matter of practical concern, rather than an academic exercise, for such differentiation will, in turn, often solve the problem of treatment versus nontreatment.

I am presenting a limited number of examples of simulated fractures that I find to pose continuing problems of differential diagnosis for my residents and for my radiologic colleagues. These nonfractures are the products of either normal variation or projection faults. They are seen in practice with sufficient frequency to be worthy of careful study and recall.

ACKNOWLEDGMENT

I wish to express my appreciation to Year Book Medical Publishers for permission to reproduce material from my book *An Atlas of Normal Roentgen Variants That May Simulate Disease.*

REFERENCE

1. Keats TE: An Atlas of Normal Roentgen Variants That May Simulate Disease. Year Book, Chicago, 1973

Theodore E. Keats, M.D.: *Professor and Chairman, Department of Radiology, University of Virginia College of Medicine, Charlottesville, Va.*

Reprint requests should be addressed to Dr. Theodore E. Keats, Department of Radiology, University of Virginia College of Medicine, Charlottesville, Va. 22901.

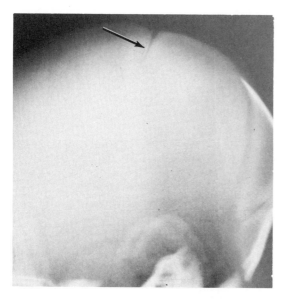

Fig. 1. Neonate with parietal fissure due to persistent strip of membranous bone matrix. These fissures, often mistaken for fracture, disappear as the child matures.

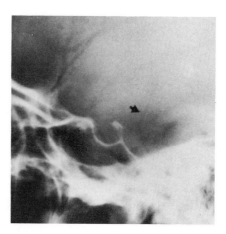

Fig. 2. Groove for the middle temporal artery simulating fracture. These are often bilateral. They are more easily identifiable as vascular grooves on stereoscopy.

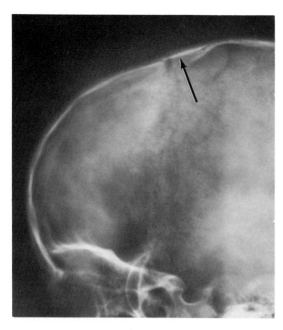

Fig. 3. Fusing anterior fontanel bone (an accessory bone) simulating fracture.

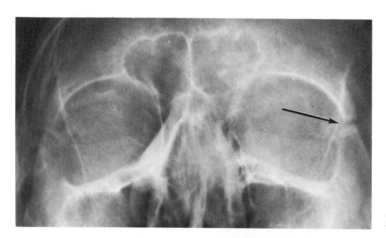

Fig. 4. Zygomaticofrontal suture, with slight rotation of the head, simulating a fracture.

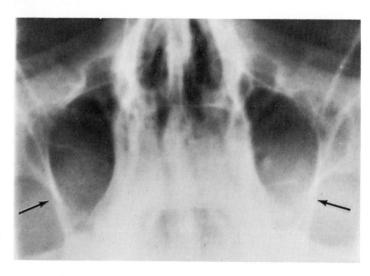

Fig. 5. Simulated fractures of the lateral wall of the maxillary antra produced by the posterior superior alveolar canals.

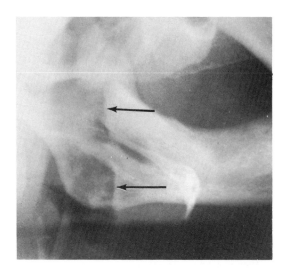

Fig. 6. Pharyngeal air shadow over the base of the tongue, superimposed on the mandible, resembling a fracture.

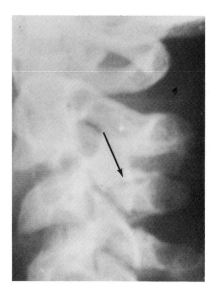

Fig. 8. Simulated fracture of the posterior neural arch of C-3 produced by rotation.

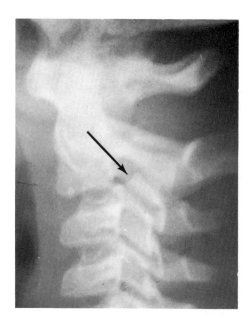

Fig. 7. Simulated fracture of the neural arch of C-3 produced by rotation. Correction of the patient's position and repetition of the examination will eliminate this shadow.

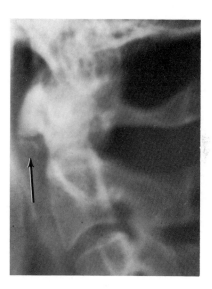

Fig. 9. The accessory ossicle of the anterior arch of C-1 may be confused with a fracture of the anterior arch.

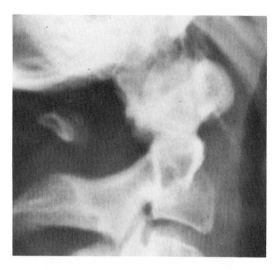

Fig. 10. Developmental absence of the laminas of C-1. Variations in development of the neural arch of C-1 are common, ranging from complete absence to absence of various portions of the arch.

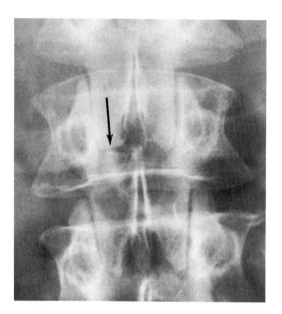

Fig. 11. Ununited ossification center of the end of the right inferior articular process of L-3, which may be mistaken for a fracture.

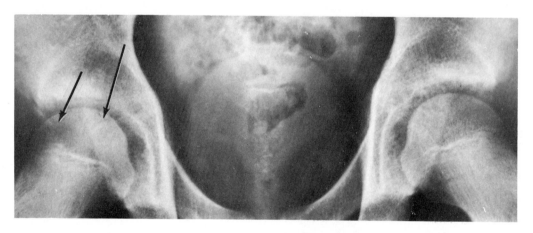

Fig. 12. Normal irregular ossification of the acetabulum in a 13-year-old boy. The unfused ossification centers may be confused with fracture, especially since they are more apparent on the right.

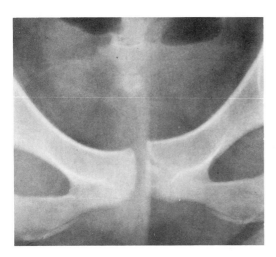

Fig. 13. Normal malalignment of the symphysis pubis in a 14-year-old girl. The lower margin of the symphysis is a more reliable indicator of proper alignment than the upper margin.

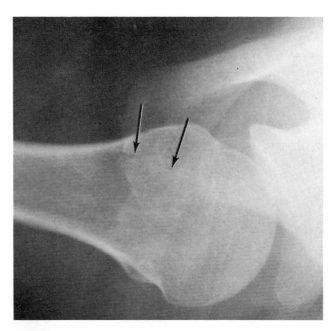

Fig. 14. The os acromiale. This secondary ossification center persists into adult life as a separate bone and is often mistaken for a fracture of the acromion process when seen in the axillary projection. It is usually bilateral.

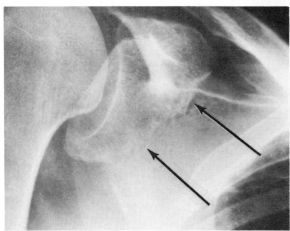

Fig. 15. Simulated fracture of the neck of the scapula produced by the prominent trabeculae frequently seen in this location.

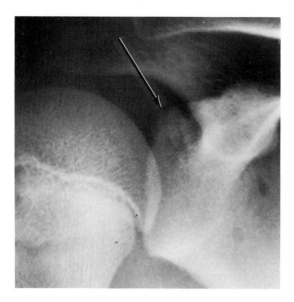

Fig. 16.   The normal irregularity of the growing glenoid process may be mistaken for fracture.

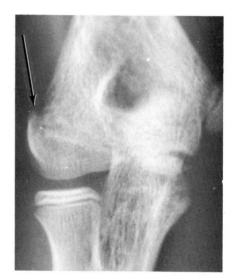

Fig. 17.   Normal offset of the capitellum in a 12-year-old boy. This apparent malalignment may be confused with traumatic displacement.

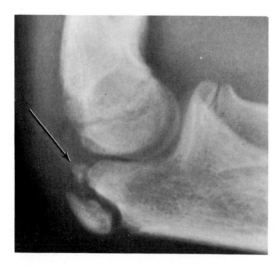

Fig. 18.   The arrow points to a separate apical nucleus of ossification for the olecranon process, not a fracture. Avulsion fractures in this area retract proximally.

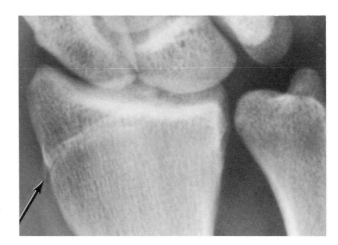

Fig. 19. The normal spurlike projection of the epiphysis at the epiphyseal line may simulate avulsion injury.

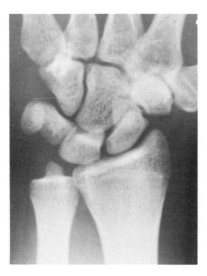

Fig. 20. Simulated fracture or rotary dislocation of the navicular produced by faulty positioning of the hand for the PA projection. Note the position of the ulnar styloid along the midline of the ulna, rather than at its lateral edge.

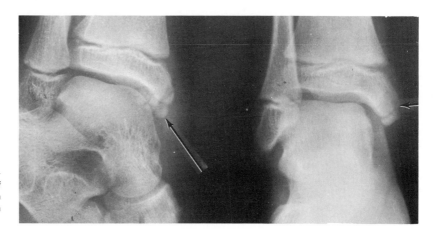

Fig. 21. The normal irregular ossification of the tip of the medial malleolus in adolescence may simulate a fracture.

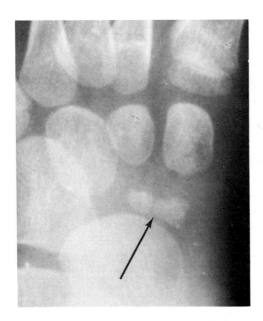

Fig. 22. Normal ossification of the tarsal navicular from duplicate irregular centers in a 6-year-old boy. Multicentric ossification should not be mistaken for a fracture.

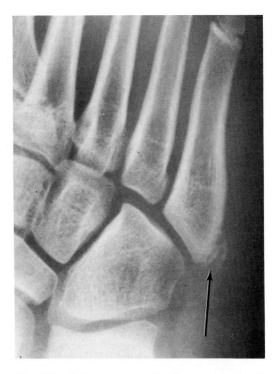

Fig. 23. Multicentric ossification centers for the tuberosity of the fifth metatarsal in a 12-year-old girl, simulating fracture.

Skull

Thomas A. Tomsick, A. Alan Chambers, and Robert R. Lukin

IT IS DIFFICULT to make an accurate determination of the incidence of skull fracture. Roberts and Shopfner[16] discovered fractures in 8.6% of 570 children who had suffered head trauma, whereas Loop and Bell[13] found fractures in 6.2% of 1500 emergency room patients examined for head trauma.

Cranial vault fractures are, of course, more easily recognized than basal skull fractures; at times it may be possible to define the latter only on base views or by use of tomography. The situation is further complicated by the fact that the patient with head-neck trauma must be placed in the potentially hazardous hyperextended position for base views.

Right and left lateral, AP, and Towne projections suffice for an initial examination series. Appropriate base or tangential films may be added as clinically indicated. Obviously, films of the highest technical quality are necessary so that fractures with clinically significant sequelae will not be missed.

Awareness of normal vascular markings, sutures, and artifacts that may masquerade radiographically as fractures is mandatory.[1,10] The chief source of difficulty is related to external carotid artery branches, which cause bony grooves that appear as linear radiolucencies. These vascular grooves are usually less lucent than fractures of the same size; they frequently have sclerotic borders, and they often branch, becoming narrower distally. Middle meningeal artery grooves involve the inner table, whereas the deep temporal branches of the internal maxillary artery, the middle temporal branch of the superficial temporal artery, and the supraorbital branch of the ophthalmic artery involve the outer table. Diploic venous channels less frequently cause confusion, since they tend to be wider and less straight than fractures, and they typically communicate with venous lakes.

The appearance of a suture varies with age. Normal sutures beyond late childhood are typically serpiginous, with sclerotic edges, and they usually present little difficulty. The sutures and fissures that repeatedly present difficulty have recently been reviewed by Allen and associates.[1] Abnormal densities due to artifacts (gas in lacerations, opacities due to foreign bodies) may be suspected on the basis of a careful examination of the soft tissues in multiple projections, and may be confirmed by physical examination of the patient's head.

Skull fractures may be linear, diastatic, comminuted, or depressed. The mechanisms of fracture production were described by Gurdjian and associates in 1953.[8] Inbending of the calvarium at the point of impact is accompanied by outbending at the periphery. If the inbending does not cause a fracture at the point of impact, the skull rebounds. Peripheral outbending may be of sufficient magnitude to cause a linear fracture that extends radially, both toward the region of impact and in the opposite direction.

A *linear* fracture appears as a lucent line with sharply defined margins. Its course may be straight, angular, or curvilinear. Because of an oblique or beveled course through the vault, a double lucency may be seen as the fracture penetrates the inner and outer tables (Fig. 1).

A fracture not initially visualized may be seen clearly on a short-term follow-up film. A sharply defined fracture may lose its well-demarcated borders and actually appear to widen slightly weeks to months following trauma. Many factors, including early resorption along the fracture margins, may be responsible for these observations. Healing occurs slowly, usually requiring 3–6 months in an infant or

Thomas A. Tomsick, M.D.: *Assistant Professor of Radiology, University of Cincinnati College of Medicine; Department of Radiology, Cincinnati General Hospital, Cincinnati, Ohio.* A. Alan Chambers, M.D.: *Assistant Professor of Radiology, University of Cincinnati College of Medicine; Department of Radiology, Cincinnati General Hospital, Veterans Adminisration Hospital, Cincinnati, Ohio.* Robert R. Lukin, M.D.: *Associate Professor of Radiology, University of Cincinnati College of Medicine; Department of Radiology, Cincinnati General Hospital, Good Samaritan Hospital, Cincinnati, Ohio.*

Reprint requests should be addressed to Dr. Thomas A. Tomsick, Department of Radiology, University of Cincinnati College of Medicine, Cincinnati General Hospital, Cincinnati, Ohio 45229.

0037-198X/78/1301-0007 $2.00/0

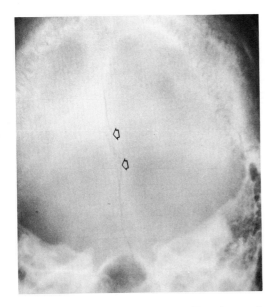

Fig. 1.   Occipital fracture with double linear lucency (arrows) due to the bevel of the fracture.

young child, 12 months in an older child, and longer in an adult.[17] During healing, new bone formation may bridge the fracture at any point, so that a discontinuous line of inhomogeneous density may result. Complete bony healing may not occur; instead, there may be fibrous tissue bridging the bony defect.

Diastasis usually implies a traumatic suture separation (Fig. 2), but it may also refer to a fracture with separated margins. In adults, diastasis frequently occurs when a fracture line extends into a suture. Isolated sutural diastasis occurs more commonly in children and young adults prior to complete suture closure (Fig. 3). Normal variations in suture width (particularly in the squamosal and lambdoid sutures) sometimes make the diagnosis of sutural diastasis difficult. However, it should be suspected when a well-defined alteration in suture width occurs, especially if it is unilateral.

Comminuted fractures result when an object strikes with great force; in such cases, the inbending results in fragmentation, with multiple radial fractures and often a *depressed* fragment. *En face,* this fracture may appear stellate (Fig. 4). Overlapping fragments of the fracture cause increased density; tangential views are necessary for an accurate assessment of the degree of depression (Fig. 5).

Although comminution accompanying depression is the rule, the ping-pong fracture of infancy is the exception. Because of the softness and resilience of the infantile calvarium, an inbend without a fracture line may occur.[7] Again, this fracture is best seen tangentially. In fact, *en face* views may be normal or may show

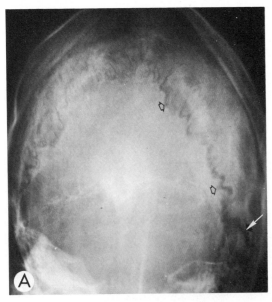
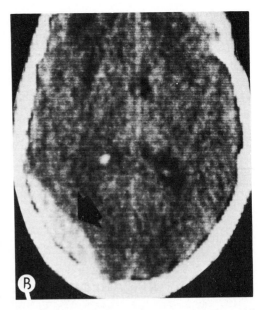

Fig. 2.   (A) Diastasis of left lambdoid suture (open arrow) and squamosal suture (white arrow) following an automobile accident. (B) CT scan shows a lens-shaped peripheral collection of blood typical of epidural hematoma (arrow).[3]

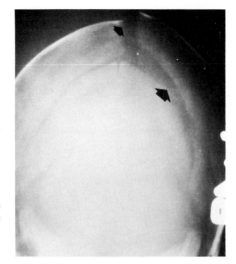

Fig. 3. Diastasis of sagittal suture (small arrow) and left lambdoid suture (large arrow) in a newborn following forceps delivery. Elevation of left parietal bone and mild depression of right parietal bone with cephalhematoma are present. (Courtesy of Dr. C. Benton, Children's Hospital Medical Center, Cincinnati, Ohio.)

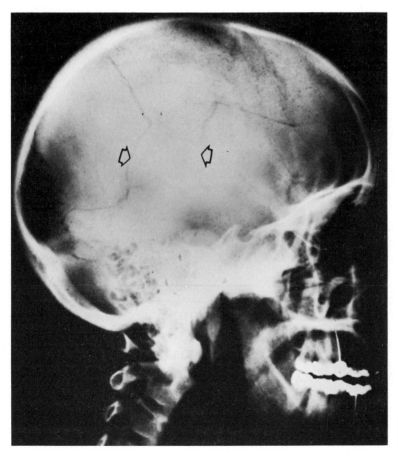

Fig. 4. Comminuted depressed fracture. Multiple fracture lines radiate from a central depressed fragment (open arrows).

29

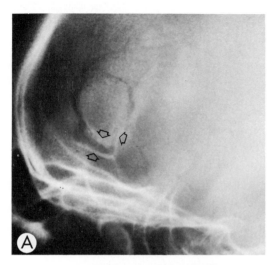

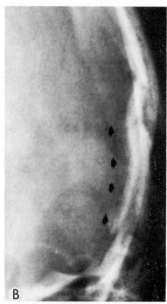

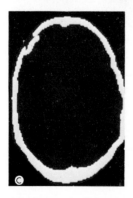

Fig. 5. Depressed comminuted fracture following hammer blow. (A) Arrows point to dense overlapping fragments. (B) Tangential fluoroscopic spot film shows 6 mm depression of central fragment (arrows). (C) CT scan (window level 100 EMI units) confirms the 6-mm depression.

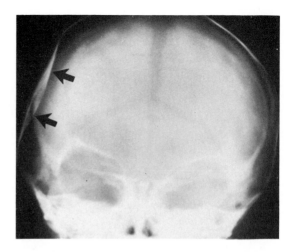

Fig. 6. Ping-pong fracture. Newborn with an inbending of the right parietal calvarium (arrows) probably due to forceps delivery. The lateral view was normal. (Courtesy of Dr. W. Smith, Riley Hospital for Children, Indiana University, Indianapolis.)

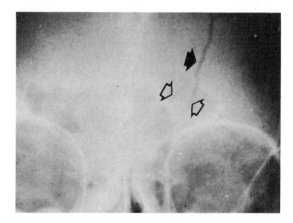

Fig. 7. Compound fracture. Linear fracture in left frontal region (solid arrow) extends to lateral margin of left frontal sinus and then divides to involve both anterior and posterior sinus walls (open arrows). Sinus is opacified.

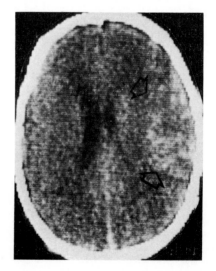

Fig. 8. CT scan. Cerebral contusion evidenced by a heterogeneous area (arrows) whose average density is higher than that of adjacent normal tissue. The higher density is due to confluent petechial extravasation of blood in swollen brain substance.

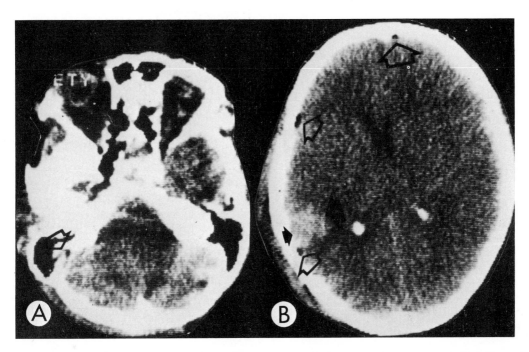

Fig. 9.   Traumatic cerebral hematoma. (A) Open arrow shows a linear fracture in posterior aspect of left petrous bone. (B) CT scan. Immediately above the fracture lies a localized region of increased density representing a posterior temporal intracerebral hematoma (closed arrows). Open arrows indicate small collections of air that entered subarachnoid space from mastoid air cells.

increased density because the depressed calvarium is viewed tangentially (Fig. 6.)

Compound fractures of the skull may be external, by virtue of communication through a skin laceration, or internal, by means of communication with a paranasal sinus or mastoid (Fig. 7).

The clinical significance of the skull fracture lies in the associated trauma to the brain and its coverings; the types of injury include the following: (1) cerebral contusion; (2) hematoma, either intracerebral, subdural, or epidural; (3) vascular occlusion, aneurysm, or arteriovenous shunt; (4) pneumocephalus; (5) infection; (6) cerebrospinal fluid (CSF) leakage; (7) cranial nerve palsies; (8) leptomeningeal cyst or enlarging skull fracture.

Cerebral contusion, intracerebral hematoma, and subdural hematoma frequently occur in the absence of fracture. However, the more severe the trauma, the greater the likelihood of these complications (Figs. 8, 9, and 10).

Epidural hematoma is a frequent sequela to a fracture extending across a meningeal vessel, usually the middle meningeal artery (Fig. 2B).

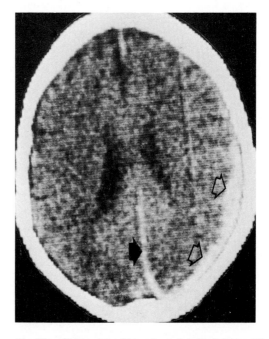

Fig. 10.   Right subdural hematoma is indicated by a thin crescentic extra-axial collection that spreads over a large portion of posterior right convexity (open arrow), as well as into the interhemispheric fissure (closed arrow).[4]

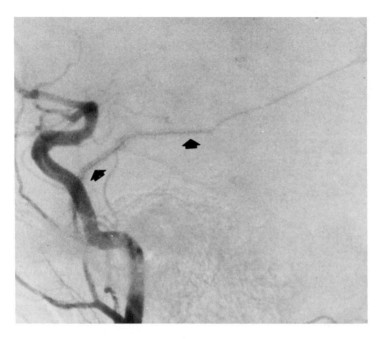

Fig. 11. Traumatic arteriovenous fistula with "railroad tracking" (arrows). The denser central posterior division of the middle meningeal artery is paralleled by meningeal venous filling.

A venous epidural hematoma may occur from a fracture crossing a dural sinus. Injury to a meningeal artery by a fracture may cause a traumatic arteriovenous fistula, which is characterized angiographically by the railroad-track appearance of early opacifying meningeal veins paralleling the opacified artery (Fig. 11). Injury to the meningeal artery also may be manifested angiographically by a false aneurysm, extravasation, or thrombosis of that vessel.

Internal carotid artery injury may result in carotid-cavernous fistula (Fig. 12), arterial rupture, true or false aneurysm, intimal damage and thrombus formation, or total occlusion.[3] Traumatic aneurysm of cortical vessels may be secondary to either closed head trauma or penetrating injury, and it is commonly associated with intracerebral hematoma (Fig. 13). These unusual aneurysms may diminish in size, disappear spontaneously, or enlarge and rupture at a later date.[2]

Internal compound fractures that involve a sinus, mastoid, or middle ear may allow air to

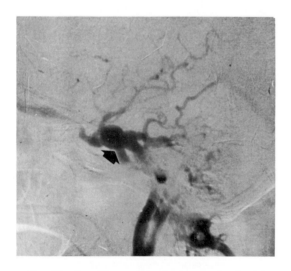

Fig. 12. Carotid-cavernous fistula associated with a comminuted fracture. Internal carotid artery flows into cavernous sinus (arrow), resulting in rapid venous shunting and scanty middle cerebral artery filling.

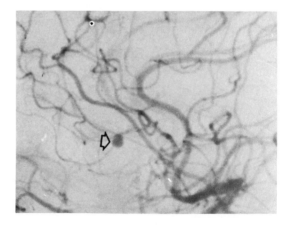

Fig. 13. Traumatic pseudoaneurysm (arrow) of a cortical branch of the middle cerebral artery that subsequently enlarged and ruptured. This was associated with a linear skull fracture and subdural hematoma.

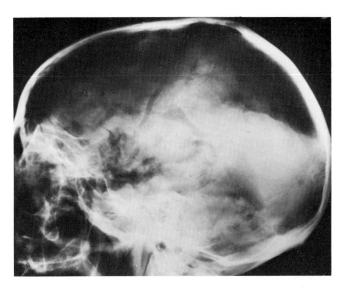

Fig. 14. Massive subdural and subarachnoid air secondary to linear frontal fracture through frontal sinus.

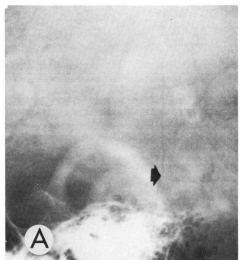

enter the subdural space, subarachnoid space, ventricles, or cerebral tissue (Fig. 9, 14).[5] Noninfected intracranial gas collections, which are usually treated conservatively, may be symptomatic and require more aggressive therapy.[14]

Osteomyelitis may complicate a compound skull fracture, as elsewhere in the body. Intracranial infection caused by compound fractures may involve the subdural, epidural, or subarachnoid spaces, or may lead to brain abscess (Fig. 15). Localized gas accumulations

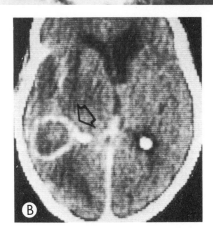

Fig. 15. (A) Linear left temporal fracture (arrow). (B) Six weeks later a left posterior temporal lobe abscess developed. This postcontrast CT scan shows a ring of enhancement (arrow) and mass effect.

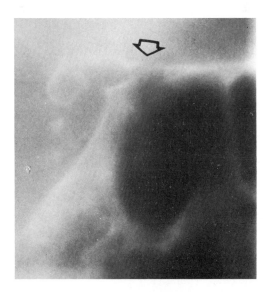

Fig. 16. Oblique polytomographic section of optic canal shows a linear fracture (arrow) associated with ipsitateral loss of vision and subsequent optic atrophy.

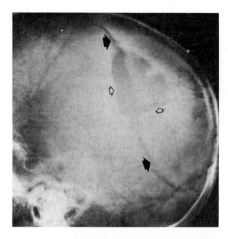

Fig. 17. Leptomeningeal cyst. This 27-month-old boy sustained a linear parietal fracture at age 12 months. The widened fracture line (closed arrows) and localized defect (open arrows) were caused by a leptomeningeal cyst (surgically proven). (Courtesy of Dr. C. Benton, Children's Hospital Medical Center, Cincinnati, Ohio.)

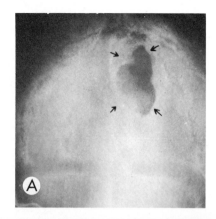

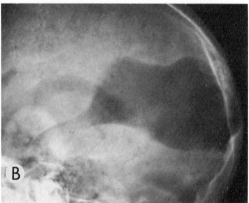

Fig. 18. Enlarging skull fracture of childhood. This 7-year-old girl fell from a third-story window at age 2 years, suffering severe neurologic deficits that subsequently improved. (A) An occipitoparietal bony defect was palpable in the region of the sharply marginated radiographic lucency (arrows). (B) Pneumoencephalogram shows porencephalic enlargement of lateral ventricle extending into the bony defect. (Courtesy of Dr. C. Benton, Children's Hospital Medical Center, Cincinnati, Ohio.)

may occur because of infection caused by a gas-forming organism.

CSF rhinorrhea and otorrhea are other complications of compound fracture. Cribriform plate fracture most commonly leads to rhinorrhea, and it may not be easy to demonstrate, even with tomography. Inspection of tomograms for localized sinus opacification may give an indirect clue to the site of origin of the leak.

Cranial nerve palsies may be secondary to compression by edematous or displaced brain (such as third nerve paresis caused by uncal herniation), or may be the result of a fracture involving a neural foramen, with local hematoma formation or direct nerve contusion (Fig. 16). The details of petrous bone fractures and subsequent seventh and eighth nerve dysfunction have been discussed in a previous *Seminar*.[15]

Not only may skull fractures fail to heal, they may actually enlarge, for a variety of reasons. Disruption of the meninges at the fracture may allow arachnoid to herniate through the dura and become anchored in the fracture. Complex adhesions and a leptomeningeal cyst may form, widen the fracture line, and cause a localized bony defect (Fig. 17).[18]

The enlarging skull fracture of childhood need not be associated with a true leptomeningeal cyst. A diastatic fracture and meningeal tear may be associated with severe local cerebral injury, resulting in ventricular enlargement or porencephaly. The porencephalic cavity transmits CSF pulsations to the fracture, resulting in enlargement (Fig. 18, 19).[11,12]

A rare form of intraosseous leptomeningeal cyst of the posterior fossa has been described wherein a fracture in the relatively thicker occipital bone is associated with an arachnoid and dural tear. The arachnoid herniation involves only the inner table and becomes trapped, and over a long period of time an intraosseous cystic collection forms (Fig. 20).[5,9]

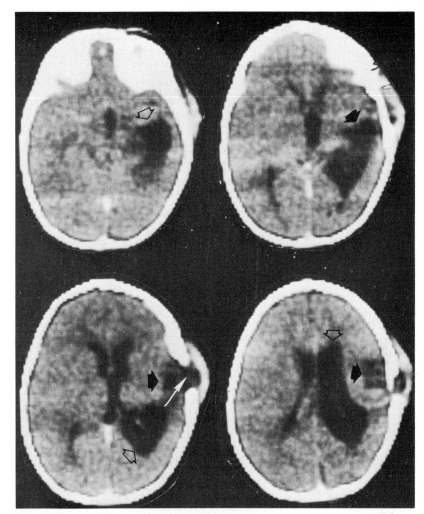

Fig. 19. Enlarging skull fracture in a 6 month old girl who sustained a diastatic fracture at 3 weeks of age. A region of low-density porencephaly (solid black arrow) of the right frontotemporal region underlies the enlarged fracture (white arrow). Ipsilateral enlargement of the right lateral ventricle, particularly its temporal horn, is evident (open arrows). Operation disclosed porencephaly and meningeal adhesions.

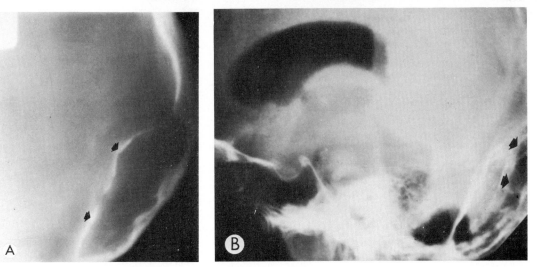

Fig. 20. Intraosseous leptomeningeal cyst. This 18-year-old student suffered a midline occipital fracture at age 2 years. (A) Midline lateral tomogram of the occipital bone shows a scalloped lesion with forward expansion of the thin inner table (arrows). (B) Brow-up pneumoencephalogram shows gas within the cystic cavity (arrows) via a communication with the cisterna magna. Surgery confirmed an intraosseous cavity. (Reproduced by permission from Dunsker and McCreary: J Neurosurg 34:687–692, 1971.)

REFERENCES

1. Allen WE, Kier EL, Rothman SL: Pitfalls in the evaluation of skull trauma. Radiol Clin North Am 11:479–503, 1973

2. Asari S, Nakamura S, Yamada O, et al: Traumatic aneurysm of peripheral cerebral arteries. J Neurosurg 46:795–803, 1977

3. Bergeron RT, Rumbaugh CL: Non space-occupying sequelae of head trauma. Radiol Clin North Am 12:315–331, 1974

4. Davis KR, Taveras JM, Roberson GH, et al: Computed tomography in head trauma. Semin Roentgenol 12:53–62, 1977

5. Dunsker SB, McCreary HS: Leptomeningeal cyst of the posterior fossa: Case report. J Neurosurg 34:687–692, 1971

6. Eaglesham DC: Radiological aspects of intracranial pneumocephalus. Br J Radiol 18:335–343, 1945

7. Genieser NB, Becker MH: Head trauma in children. Radiol Clin North Am 12:333–342, 1974

8. Gurdjian ES, Webster JE, Lissner HR: Observations on prediction of fracture site in head trauma. Radiology 60:226–235, 1953

9. Hillman RSL, Kieffer SA, Ortiz H, et al: Intraosseous leptomeningeal cysts of the posterior cranial fossa. Radiology 116:655–659, 1975

10. Keats TE: An Atlas of Normal Roentgen Variants That May Simulate Disease. Chicago, Year Book, 1973, pp 5–65

11. Lende RA: Enlarging skull fractures of childhood. Neuroradiology 7:119–124, 1974

12. Lende RA, Erickson TC: Growing skull fractures of childhood. J Neurosurg 18:479–489, 1961

13. Loop JW, Bell RS: The utility and futility of radiographic skull examination for trauma. N Engl J Med 284:236–239, 1971

14. Markham JW: The clinical features of pneumocephalus based upon a survey of 284 cases with report of 11 additional cases. Acta Neurochir 16:1–78, 1967

15. Potter GD: Trauma to the temporal bone. Semin Roentgenol 4:143–150, 1969

16. Roberts FR, Shopfner CE: Plain skull roentgenograms in children with head trauma. Am J Roentgenol 114:230–240, 1972

17. Taveras JM, Wood EH: Diagnostic Neuroradiology. Baltimore, Williams & Wilkins, 1976, pp 1054–1058

Face

Kenneth D. Dolan and Charles G. Jacoby

THE maxillofacial skeleton is very vulnerable to injury. Even though it is padded by overlying skin, fat, and muscles of expression, the face consists of rather thin and poorly supported bone that can easily break under the force of a blow. Also, the face seems to be a favored target in fights.

On analyzing 323 facial features, Nakamura and Gross[8] found that 59% of their patients were injured by intended violence; automobile accidents produced the injuries in 17%, and miscellaneous causes such as other accidents, falls, and sports accounted for the remaining 24%. Of their 323 patients, 75% were in the 10–40-year age group.

The form that a given injury assumes depends on several factors. These include the contact point or area on the face and the velocity and shape of the injuring object. Generally, an object with a small surface area traveling at a velocity sufficient to produce injury will produce only local injury. High-velocity contact between the face and an object with a large surface area produces more extensive (usually comminuted) local injury, together with propagation of the fracture to other parts of the face. This variety of fracture is common in connection with automobile accidents.

Radiologic evaluation of facial fractures requires comprehensive knowledge of maxillofacial anatomy, well-positioned films taken from views chosen to illustrate pertinent facial anatomy, and an understanding of the patterns of facial injury.

MAXILLOFACIAL VIEWS AND RADIOLOGIC ANATOMY

Merrell and associates[7] detailed the radiologic anatomy of each standard maxillofacial view.* Our presentation will emphasize key anatomic areas represented on the standard maxillofacial views.

In the patient suspected of having facial injury, it must be emphasized that the coned-down views customarily obtained for paranasal sinus disease are not adequate to evaluate the entire maxillofacial skeleton. We routinely use 25 × 30 cm film with a cone large enough to include the skull, maxillofacial, and mandibular areas in a single frame. Stereoscopic views may be helpful to those accustomed to their use.

The Waters and Caldwell views should be made as posteroanterior (PA) projections for the clearest representation of maxillofacial features. We ordinarily delay definitive filming until the patient can cooperate for PA views, unless the patient cannot assume the sitting position.

Waters View

The Waters view gives the best representation of the midface. Proper positioning is indicated when the alveolar border of the maxilla lies just above the surface of the petrous bone.

Three imaginary lines of bony continuity are evident on the Waters view (Fig. 1). Beginning at the inner surface of the zygomaticofrontal suture on either side, the first line (A in Fig. 1) follows the orbital surface of the zygoma, the orbital surface of the maxilla, the frontal process of the maxilla, and the arch produced by the nasal bones; it is continuous with the same features on the opposide side. This resembles a pair of half-frame reading glasses.

The second line of continuity (B) begins at the outer surface of the zygomaticomaxillary suture, continues downward along the orbital process of the zygoma and along the upper border of the zygomatic arch, and curves medially to the glenoid fossa of the temporomandibular joint. This line is present on both sides.

The third line (C) begins at the root of the zygoma, extends along the inferior border of the

---

*These articles have been collected into a single volume and are available from the American Academy of Ophthalmology and Otolaryngology, Rochester, Minn. 55901.

Kenneth D. Dolan, M.D.: *Professor;* Charles G. Jacoby, M.D.: *Assistant Professor; Department of Radiology, The University of Iowa Hospitals and Clinics, Iowa City, Iowa.*

Reprint requests should be addressed to Dr. Kenneth D. Dolan, Department of Radiology, The University of Iowa Hospitals and Clinics, Iowa City, Iowa 52242.

© *1978 by Grune & Stratton, Inc.*

0037-198X/78/1301-0004 $2.00/0

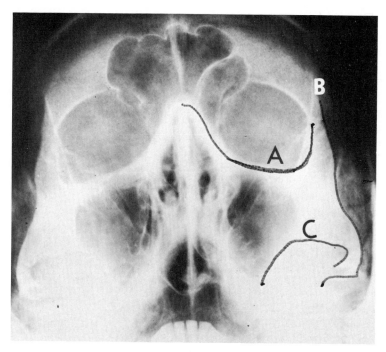

Fig. 1. Standard Waters view with lines of continuity (see text).

zygomatic arch, and follows the lateral border of the maxilla to the dentoalveolar margin. This line is also paired.

Lines B and C together outline an area resembling the side view of the elephant's head and trunk. The three lines of continuity are illustrated in Fig. 1.

In the Waters view, one may also assess maxillary sinus size and transparency, the posterior portion of the orbital floor, and the location of the infraorbital canal.

Caldwell View

The ideal projection for the Caldwell view places the floor of the orbit just above the surface of the petrous bone and reveals the upper portion of the maxillary sinuses. The frontal region, orbits, superior orbital fissures, and orbital floors can be visualized above the petrous bones (Fig. 2). The maxillary alveolus and upper dental arch may be visualized below the petrous bone.

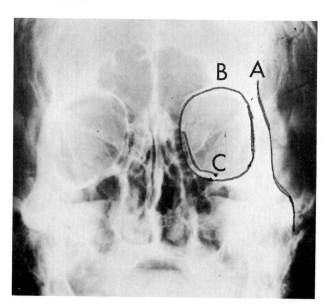

Fig. 2. Standard Caldwell view with lines of continuity (see text).

A line of continuity (A in Fig. 2) along the orbital process of the frontal bone, the outer surface of the orbital process of the zygoma, and the zygomatic arch can be followed to where it disappears over the mastoid process of the temporal bone.

Each orbit can be evaluated in this projection. Starting at the inner margin of the zygomaticomaxillary suture, a line continues upward along the roof of the orbit to the superomedial quadrant of the orbit (B). The palpable margin of the orbit, which lies below the roof, can be seen in the upper outer orbital quadrant. Below the frontal sinus, the cortical margin of the orbit divides into two parallel lines. The medial line is produced by the posterior lacrimal crest and continues laterally along the plane of the anterior orbital floor to merge with the inner surface of the orbital process of the zygoma. The lateral line (C) along the medial orbit is produced by a portion of the ethmoidal lamina papyracea and is continuous with the more posterior orbital floor surface. It can be followed laterally to the inferior orbital fissure. Often a notch produced by the infraorbital neurovascular structures will be seen in the distal part of this cortical line.

Centrally in this view, lamina dura margins of the frontal sinus can be traced bilaterally. The transparency of the sinuses should be compared with that of the orbital cavity. These areas of transparency are normally about equal.

The nasal bones nearly parallel the plane of the film in this view and are not visualized. The pyramidal nasal aperture is well seen between the maxillary sinuses. Superiorly the frontal process of the maxilla, and inferiorly the medial border of the maxilla surround the nasal fossa. Centrally the perpendicular plate of the ethmoid and the vomer form a bony septum that ends at the hard palate.

A transverse cortical line crosses the upper orbit. Laterally it begins at the zygomaticofrontal suture and represents the junction of the frontal and sphenoidal orbital surfaces. Medially the line represents the cerebral surface of the lesser sphenoidal wing. In the midline, it represents the roof of the sphenoidal sinuses. The oblique superior orbital fissure can be seen below the lesser sphenoidal wing. The oblique orbital line (innominate line) can be seen as a vertical cortical line merging with the outer portion of the transverse orbital line. This line is produced by the orbital process of the sphenoidal bone.

General orientation of the orbital and maxillary height should be evaluated on this view. Ordinarily the vertical height of the orbit equals that of the maxillary sinus.

Basal View

The basal projection can be obtained either with the patient in a prone position, using a vertex-submental beam, or with the patient in the upright position with neck extended, using a submental-vertex beam. The information provided is essentially the same with either method. The ideal basal view is one in which the mandibular symphysis is superimposed on the frontal sinus. A hyperextended basal view has been used to evaluate the frontal sinus surfaces. In this view, the symphysis is projected in front of the frontal sinuses.

If the basal projection is underexposed, the zygomatic arches will be well seen laterally (Fig. 9B). An exposure adequate for central features usually overexposes the zygomatic arches but does allow a view of the lateral orbital surface, the posterior maxillary sinus surface, and the sphenoidal surface of the temporal fossa. Whalen and Berne described these three key lines.[10]

The basal view also allows evaluation of the relationship between the mandibular condyle and the glenoid fossa of the temporomandibular joint. Centrally, the ethmoidal and sphenoidal sinuses can be visualized. The transparent ethmoidal sinus has many visible bony septa. If blood is present, the sinus becomes opaque and the septa disappear. Blood in the nasal fossa or enlargement of the nasal turbinates may make the ethmoidal sinus appear less transparent, but the septa will remain visible.

Lateral View

The lateral view is obtained by convention as a left lateral, with the central beam in the axis of the pupil and centered over the temporal fossa. The ideal projection has nearly perfect superimposition of the two mandibular rami, as well as the sphenoidal surfaces of the temporal fossae.

The lateral view allows evaluation of the

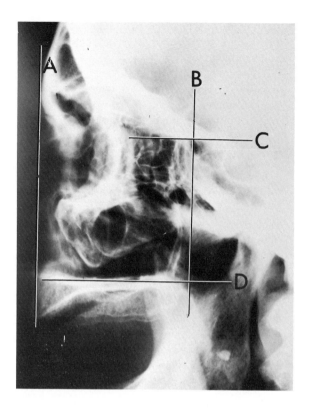

Fig. 3. Lateral view with vertical and horizontal position lines (see text).

frontal surface of the skull, the anterior and posterior surfaces of the midline of the frontal sinuses, the height of the orbits and maxillary sinuses, and the positions of the maxillary and mandibular dental arches. The posterior surface of the maxillary sinuses and at least the anterior surface of the pterygoid processes of the sphenoid can be evaluated in the region of the pterygomaxillary fissures.

Figure 3 illustrates several important relationships. An anterior vertical line connecting the frontal sinus surface and anterior hard palate (A) should parallel a posterior vertical line connecting the sphenoidal wing and posterior edge of the hard palate (B). Also, a horizontal line paralleling the planum sphenoidale (C) should parallel the nasal cavity surface of the hard palate (D). Alterations in these lines may be caused by displacement of the palate and facial structures and should suggest a LeFort injury, but they may also occur in patients with maxillofacial developmental defects.

We prefer a coned underexposed lateral view to assess the nasal bones and anterior maxillary spine.

Panoramic Facial Views

The Panorex, Orthopantomograph, and similar radiographic machines may be used to obtain panoramic views of the mandible and facial structures. While they are excellent for mandibular views, especially now that the Tomorex device is available for horizontal panoramic views, information regarding the facial structures only complements that obtained with standard radiographic views.

Supplementary Views

The PA view helps in ethmoidal roof evaluation when central facial injury is accompanied by cerebrospinal fluid rhinorrhea. This projection also allows a supplementary view of the ethmoidal surface of the orbit in the evaluation of ethmoidal fractures.

Oblique views of the lateral orbital walls have been described by Lame and Redick.[5] While separation of a lateral wall fracture may be more apparent on oblique views, the fracture is usually quite apparent on standard views.

Optic canal views are used to supplement

standard studies when signs of retrobulbar hemorrhage or visual disturbance accompany an injury. The superior orbital fissure, lesser sphenoidal wing, ethmoidal sinus, and optic canal are visualized on this projection.

Tomography

Tomographic study of facial structures has been revolutionized by the development of pleurodirectional thin-section tomography. With linear tomography, parasite shadows may obscure a fracture line. With the more complete blurring of pleurodirectional tomography, even fine fractures or those obscured by overlapping structures can be assessed. We consider tomography to be the best means of completely evaluating fractures, particularly the orbital blowout fracture. Computerized tomography has yet to be evaluated for orbital injury.

FRAGMENT ANALYSIS OF FACIAL INJURIES

Most facial fractures produce one or more fragments separated from their normal surrounding attachments. The surgical information needed from radiologic examination concerns the location of fragments and whether they are stable or need repositioning and surgical fixation. Information regarding impaction of a fragment is also important. Palpable distortion of the bones may be obscured by overlying swelling, laceration, or hematoma.

In a facial fracture, comminution of bone usually occurs at the site of impact. Thus, on radiographs, the impact usually has occurred at the site of the multiple fragments. Propagation of the stress to nearby parts of the maxillofacial skeleton may result in a shearing fracture, with separation of a large fragment of bone remote from the impact site. This occurs commonly in the LeFort injury patterns.

By evaluating the key anatomic areas described earlier, one may reconstruct the principal fragment and assess its displacement from the surrounding normal bony structures.

ROENTGEN SIGNS OF INJURY

Both suggestive and definitive signs of injury may be present in a given fracture. Generally, indirect signs are those that may also be present in other conditions, such as inflammatory or neoplastic paranasal sinus disease.

Soft-tissue swelling in the malar, nasofrontal, or periocular regions is commonly associated with maxillofacial injury. A paranasal sinus may show an air-fluid level, mucous membrane thickening, or complete opacity. In the injured patient, these signs suggest the need for careful analysis of the surrounding bones.

Subcutaneous facial air or periocular air is virtually diagnostic of a fracture in the region of a paranasal sinus. However, in the case of ethmoidal fractures, there may be no other direct evidence of the fracture on plain films. The periocular air is a strong enough indication to go directly to polytomography to locate the ethmoidal fracture. Similarly, intracranial air strongly suggests a fracture in the frontal, ethmoidal, or sphenoidal area.

Direct signs are reliable bony changes indicative of a fracture. The most common direct sign is separation of a cortical line. Displacement of a fragment may produce an area of increased absorption of x-rays where the fragment overlaps surrounding normal bone.

Merrell and associates described a useful sign of maxillofacial injury called the *abnormal linear density.*[6] A fragment of bone normally lying parallel to the film plane may be turned on edge as a result of the injury and may produce a cortical absorption line not normally present in the area. This sign, in our experience, has greatest application in injuries around the maxilla and orbital floor.

TYPES OF FRACTURES

The fragment produced by a facial injury assumes a configuration appropriate to the force and direction of the blow and the area struck by the object. Local fractures are produced by low-energy force application. More complex fractures result from larger applications of force, and culminate in high-force injuries associated with all motor vehicle accidents, producing the LeFort or "smash" injury patterns.

Local Fractures

Fractures about the frontal sinus may be difficult to recognize unless one uses both the Caldwell and lateral views. In Figure 4, the

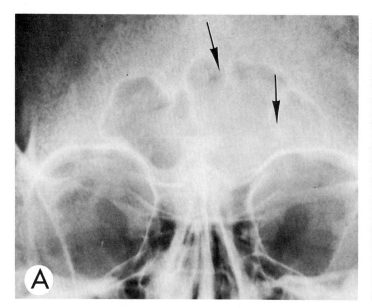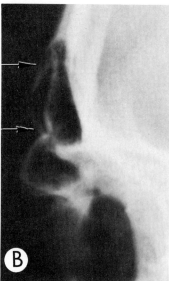

Fig. 4.   Fracture of anterior wall of frontal sinus. (A) Caldwell view with arrows at fracture lines. (B) Lateral view showing indentation of the anterior surface (arrows).

Caldwell view shows slight decrease in the frontal sinus transparency and two separation lines (arrows) extending across the sinuses. The lateral view (Fig. 4B) reveals an indentation of the anterior sinus wall resulting from a local fracture. Tomography may be necessary to evaluate the posterior surface of the injured frontal bone.

The superior orbital rim may also be injured by a local blow. Shearing of the upper rim may occur if the impact is lateral; the fragment produced may include a part of the frontal sinus margin if the impact is medial. Figure 5 illustrates two fragments separated from the

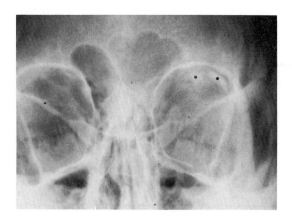

Fig. 5.   Local orbital rim fragments (dots) on Caldwell view.

upper anterior orbital margin. The more medial fragment is located at the site of the trochlear sling of the superior oblique ocular muscle. The trochlea was detached from underlying bone with this fragment.

Nasal fractures may exist independently or as part of a more extensive injury. The surgeon is primarily interested in the cosmetic appearance of the nose and restoration of nasal function after injury. Unfortunately, it is difficult to evaluate either of these aspects radiographically. In Figure 6A, interruption of the nasal arch is difficult to appreciate, although the interrupted cortical line is well visualized through the area of nasal soft-tissue swelling. Generally, nasal fractures oriented in the AP plane will interrupt the cortical line of the nasal arch in the Waters view. Transversely oriented fractures and fractures of the tip of the nasal bone are best shown in the lateral soft-tissue view (Fig. 6B).

A fracture located in the region of the lower orbital rim may simulate a blowout fracture. Figure 7 illustrates a patient who was struck along the right lower orbital border. The malar soft-tissue margin is swollen, and a defect in the cortical border of the maxillary orbital margin is present. The fragment is displaced downward and is rotated so that there is loss of the outline of the infraorbital foramen. Other views, includ-

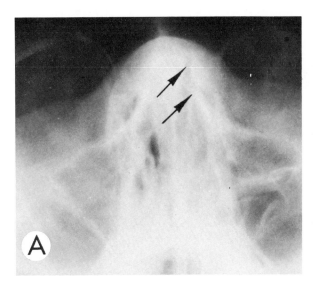
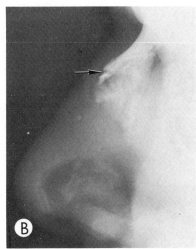

Fig. 6.   Nasal fractures. (A) Waters view showing an arch fracture. (B) Transverse separation line (arrow) and depressed tip fragment in a different patient.

ing tomography, revealed only an orbital rim injury that included a small portion of the adjacent orbital floor. Hypesthesia of the anterior cheek accompanied the fracture.

With the orbital blowout fracture, the fragment is usually limited to the maxillary surface of the orbit. By definition, the fracture excludes interruption of the orbital rim. While the mechanism of the blowout fracture has been variously explained, the major cause seems to be compression of the orbital content by a curved object so that the bony orbital floor with orbital fat herniates into the maxillary sinus. Fujino recently demonstrated experimentally the production of the blowout fracture by force

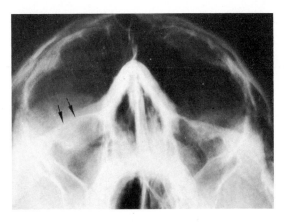

Fig. 7.   Local inferior orbital rim fracture (arrows): The fragment is displaced inferiorly. Waters view.

applied over the lower orbital rim, and related the injury to a direct compression force.[4] We agree with Emery and associates, who described injuries by the fist as being the most common cause of blowout fractures.[3] They also noted a high frequency (24%) of serious injuries to ocular structures associated with this injury. We have concluded that a blow to both ocular and orbital portions is the most likely cause of this injury.

Both the Waters and the Caldwell views are necessary to define a blowout fracture (Fig. 8). The Waters projection illustrates the integrity of the orbital rim and may show displacement of the posterior floor. The Caldwell projection often illustrates the actual floor defect. In Figure 8, a maxillary sinus soft-tissue mass is also visible on both projections. Blowout fractures may require tomographic evaluation if the floor is only slightly altered; according to Crikelair and associates, it is the definitive diagnostic technique if only suggestive findings are present on plain films.[1]

Blowout fractures are associated with a similar injury to the ethmoidal surface of the orbit in 20%–40% of patients. The medial (ethmoidal) wall is seldom injured alone. Opacity of the anterior ethmoidal area should suggest involvement here, but tomography is necessary to confirm medial injury. Ethmoidal injury may also accompany nasal fractures; this combina-

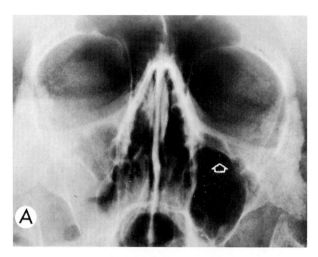

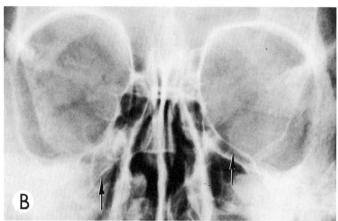

Fig. 8. Right orbital blowout fracture. (A) Waters view with normal posterior orbital floor cortical line (arrow) on the left. The orbital floor line is not seen on the right and a large soft-tissue mass projects into the maxillary sinus. (B) The Caldwell view shows a normal left orbital posterior floor line (higher arrow) and caudal displacement of the floor on the right (lower arrow).

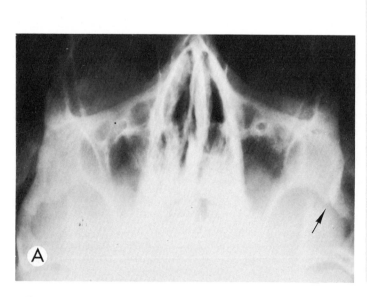

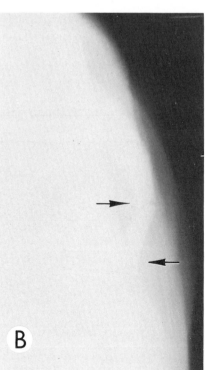

Fig. 9. Left zygomatic arch fracture shown on (A) Waters view (arrow) and (B) soft-tissue basal view. Arrows indicate the depressed zygomatic arch.

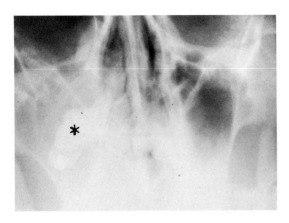

Fig. 10. Local right maxillary alveolus fracture with teeth-containing fragment (*) rotated upward into the maxillary sinus.

tion will be considered in the sections on complex fractures and the LeFort injuries.

Lateral orbital wall injury seldom occurs as a solitary fracture; it is usually associated with zygomatic complex injuries, which will be discussed later.

The zygomatic arch is another promontory susceptible to local injury. Interruption of this structure is best visualized on the Waters projection, in which interruption or overlap of fragments is usually visible (Fig. 9A). An underexposed basal projection (Fig. 9B) will confirm the presence of this fracture.

The maxillary alveolus and dental structures are also vulnerable to injury. In Figure 10, a Waters projection illustrates an avulsion fracture of the alveolus containing lateral incisor, canine, and first premolar teeth. The fragment has rotated upward along with a portion of the nasal maxillary margin into the anterior surface

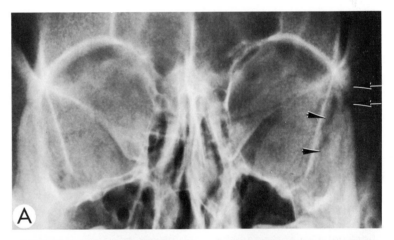

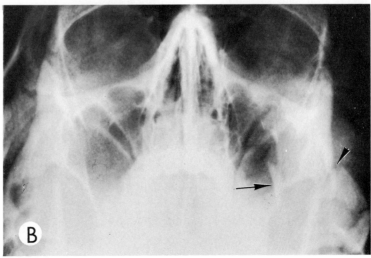

Fig. 11. Left tripod fracture. (A) Caldwell view with zygomaticofrontal suture separation (arrows). The lateral orbital wall separation is visible (arrowheads) paralleling the oblique orbital line. The zygomatic fragment is displaced downward and medially. (B) Waters view showing the zygomatic arch interruption (arrowheads). The arrow points to an abnormal linear density at the site of the lateral maxillary wall fracture. The patient was unable to open his mouth.

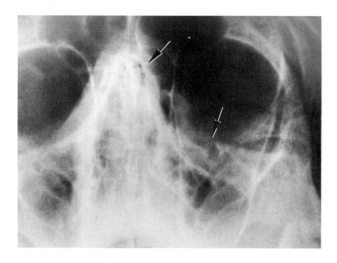

Fig. 12. Maxillary frontal process fracture (between the arrows). Note the medial displacement of the fragment, as compared to the opposite side.

of the sinus, which is filled with blood. Mandibular injury frequently accompanies such maxillary alveolar injuries, but it was not present in this patient.

Complex Fractures

The fractures in the complex category are associated with larger fragment components, or they may cross anatomic regions to produce a fragment that includes two or more anatomic parts.

The zygomaticomaxillary complex fractures have been given a variety of names: *tripod, trimalar, malar eminence,* and others. We prefer the term *tripod* fracture. The fracture results from a blow over the malar eminence that separates the zygomatic fragment from its frontal, temporal, and maxillary attachments.

The tripod fracture consists of separation of the frontal and zygomatic orbital processes, usually at the suture. Separation of the thin zygomatic surface of the lateral orbital wall extends to the region of the inferior orbital fissure. Both of these changes are best defined in the Caldwell view (Fig. 11A).

The zygomatic arch interruption may consist of a single fracture line or a comminuted interruption, as seen in the Waters projection. Separation of the zygomaticomaxillary junction may occur anywhere along the lower orbital border and lateral maxillary wall. In Figure 11B, the zygoma has been driven medially into the maxilla. The interruption along the orbital rim is barely visible, whereas a large abnormal linear density denotes the fracture of the lateral maxillary wall. Although this particular frac-

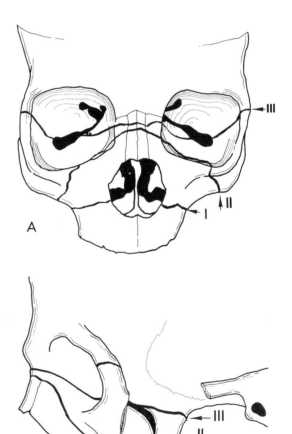

Fig. 13. LeFort weakness lines. Frontal (A) and lateral (B) drawings with the planes of weakness delimited. The zygomatic arch has been omitted in B.

ture was stable, the surgeon elected to elevate the body of the zygoma because of the flattened malar eminence resulting from the injury. Stabilization was produced with a wire suture in the zygomaticofrontal suture area and along the orbital rim. Complications of the tripod fracture include inability to open or close the mouth because of entrapment of the mandibular coronoid process by the depressed zygoma.

Fracture of the medial aspect of the maxilla in the area of the frontal process is usually accompanied by a nasal fracture. Figure 12 illustrates such a fracture in which the nasal arch is comminuted and the orbital process and medial maxilla are driven into the nasal fossa. An orbital rim step-off can be seen medial to the infraorbital canal.

It is important to recognize these fractures for several reasons. Nasal cosmetic appearance and function are disturbed. The lacrimal canal is often obstructed, producing epiphora, and the medial canthal ligament may be separated, resulting in a cosmetic deformity of the medial portion of the lids.

LeFort Fractures

The LeFort injuries are named after a French investigator who studied induced injuries and devised a system of lines representing weak facial supporting areas through which facial fractures may occur. LeFort's papers have been translated and published in a monograph available through The University of Texas at Houston.[9]

The facial skeleton is a boxlike cantilever that projects from the base of the skull below the anterior and middle cranial fossae. Centrally, the ethmoidal bones, the perpendicular plate of the ethmoid, and the vomer support the face. Laterally, the frontal and zygomatic plates of the orbit connect the maxillary sinuses to the skull. Posteriorly, the pterygoid processes of the sphenoid bone provide maxillary support. Inferiorly, the hard palate stabilizes the maxillary bones. LeFort described three areas of weakness in the facial cantilever that may be interrupted by lateral or frontal application of force (Fig. 13).

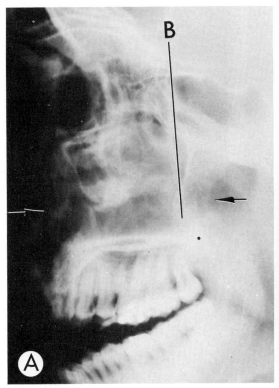
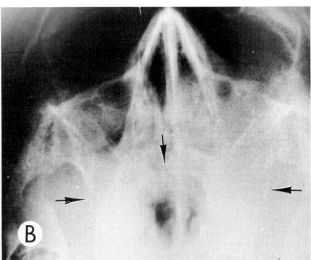

Fig. 14. LeFort I fracture. (A) Lateral view with pterygoid process fracture (posterior arrow) and anterior maxillary comminution (anterior arrow). The hard palate is displaced posteriorly, and an anterior open bite is present. (B) Waters view. The lateral arrows show the fracture plane. The vertical arrow indicates a longitudinal palate fracture.

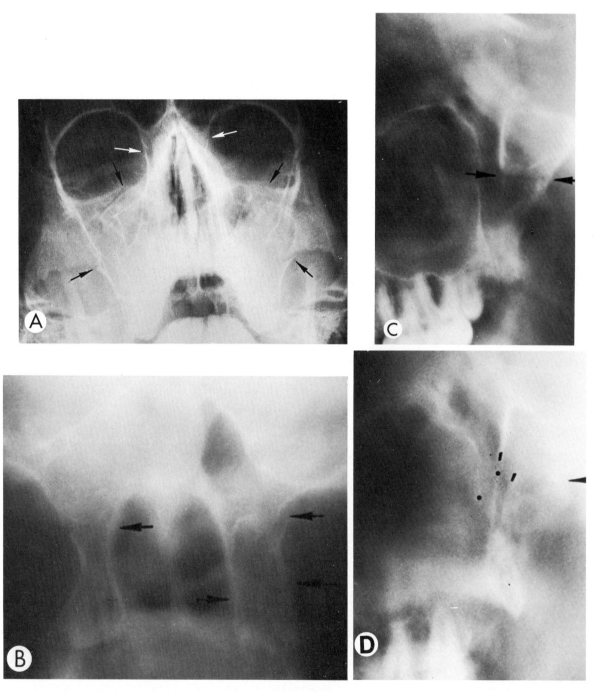

Fig. 15. LeFort II fracture. (A) Waters view. Arrows indicate the margins of the fragment. (B) Coronal tomogram showing pterygoid process fractures (arrows). (C) Right lateral tomogram showing fracture plane (arrows). (D) Left lateral tomogram. A large fracture fragment is shown (arrow). The posterior maxillary fracture (small dots) and pterygoid fracture (small bands) are demonstrated.

The first line of weakness is through the mid-portion of the maxilla and the pterygoid plates. This area is usually injured by an anterior or lateral blow to the premaxilla area. Figure 14 illustrates the LeFort I fracture. The lateral view shows pterygoid plate interruption, which is present in all types of LeFort injuries. It also shows comminution of the anterior maxillary area. An anterior open bite, in which the molars are approximated and the incisors vertically separated, is present; the hard palate is slightly displaced posteriorly behind the B line.

The Waters view shows fractures of the lateral maxillary walls, medial maxillary walls, nasal pyramidal borders, and vomer. A longitudinal palate fracture is also present. A coincidental local fracture of the left inferior orbital rim is present, but it is not a direct part of the LeFort I injury. Clinically, the lower maxillary fragments could be moved in relation to surrounding bone.

The second line of weakness described by LeFort extends across the central face in a pyramidal fashion. After a blow in the nasofrontal area, separation crosses the ethmoidal bone obliquely, extends across the medial maxillary surface of the orbit, and shears obliquely through the lateral maxilla between the inferior orbital fissure and the lateral maxillary wall. Figure 15 illustrates the appearance of a LeFort II fracture. In the Waters view, the central pyramidal separated fragment is evident. The coronal tomogram shows bilateral pterygoid process fractures, which are further illustrated in the lateral tomograms.

The third line of weakness begins in the naso-frontal area and extends across the ethmoid bone posterior to the inferior orbital fissure and pterygoid processes, then laterally through the zygomatic process of the orbits and zygomatic arches. Figure 16 illustrates a fracture through the LeFort III line of weakness, with caudal displacement of the facial fragment from the cranial base. Marked vertical elongation of the orbital shadow results from this displacement.

In our experience, one seldom finds a simple LeFort II or III injury. Combinations of one fragment on one side and a dissimilar fragment on the other lead to intermediate classification of LeFort I and II, II and III, or I and III fractures. In Figure 17a, comminuted fracture is seen in the frontal-ethmoid axis in the Caldwell view. In the Waters view, a tripod fracture has been opened laterally on the right and constitutes one facial fragment. Wide separation has occurred through the LeFort II axis on that side. On the left, there is a fracture through the zygomaticofrontal suture and zygomatic arch. The left orbital rim is intact inferiorly. This injury has produced a large facial fragment through the LeFort II line on the right and the LeFort III line on the left, with vertical rotation of the fragment, resulting in approximation of the maxillary and mandibular molars on the right and separation on the left.

The greatest confusion occurs during analysis

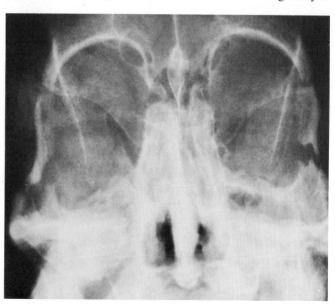

Fig. 16. LeFort III fracture. There is caudal displacement of the face from the cranial base. The orbits appear elongated.

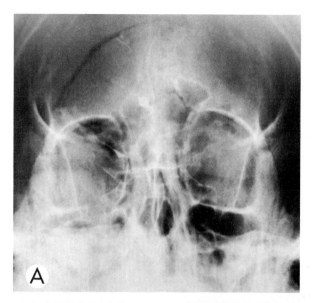

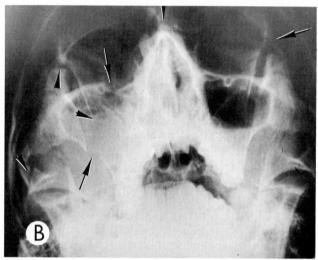

Fig. 17. Frontal-nasal-ethmoidal "smash" injury. (A) Caldwell view. (B) Waters view. Left LeFort III fracture and right LeFort II fracture are outlined by arrows. Rotation of the large fragment produced approximation of the molars on the right. A right tripod fragment is present (arrowheads).

Table 1. Frequency of Maxillofacial Fractures and Fractures Elsewhere

Type	Total	Number with Associated Fractures
Local	14	5 (30%)
Tripod	60	16 (27%)
(tripod and LeFort I)	1	
LeFort I	23	9 (40%)
(LeFort I and II)	3	
LeFort II	25	16 (64%)
(LeFort II and III)	12	6 (50%)
LeFort III	7	3 (40%)
Smash injury	6	2 (33%)
	156	51 (33%)

of those injuries in which all of the facial bones are interrupted and comminuted into many small fragments. These we classify as *central facial smash* injuries. The usual smash injuries are associated with extensive frontal bone injury, anterior cranial fossa injury, and often middle cranial fossa injury.

ASSOCIATED FRACTURES

Table 1 summarizes fractures associated with facial injuries, as detailed by Dolan.[2] Almost one-third of the entire group of facial injuries was associated with fractures elsewhere. An associated mandibular fracture was present in 23% and cranial fractures in 14%. These were most common among the LeFort and smash injuries (12 of 22). Only 2% had cervical spine injuries, and nearly one-third had peripheral skeletal or lower spine injuries.

REFERENCES

1. Crikelair GF, Rein JM, Potter GD, et al: A critical look at the "blow-out" fracture. Plast Reconstr Surg 49:374–379, 1972

2. Dolan KD: Fracturas maxilofaciales. Rev Mexicana de Radiol 25:89–103, 1971

3. Emery JM, Noorden GK, Sclernitzauer DA: Orbital floor fractures: Long-term follow-up of cases with and without surgical repair. Trans Am Acad Ophthalmol Otolaryngol 75:802–812, 1971

4. Fujino T: Experimental "blow-out" fracture of the orbit. Plast Reconstr Surg 54:81–82, 1974

5. Lame EL, Redick TJ: A new radiographic technique for fractures of the orbit and maxilla. Am J Roentgenol 127:473–480, 1976

6. Merrell RA Jr, Yanagisawa E, Smith HW: Abnormal linear density. A useful x-ray sign in the evaluation of maxillofacial fractures. Arch Otolaryngol 90:140–147, 1969

7. Merrell RA Jr, Yanagisawa E, Smith HW, Thaler S: Radiographic anatomy of the paranasal sinuses. I. Waters view. II. Lateral view. Arch Otolaryngol 87:88–99, 100–113, 1968

8. Nakumura T, Gross CW: Facial fractures. Analysis of five years of experience. Arch Otolaryngol 97:288–290, 1973

9. Tilson HB, McFee AS, Soudah HP: The Maxillofacial Works of Rene LeFort. Houston, The University of Texas Dental Branch, 1972 (PO Box 20068, Houston, Texas 77025)

10. Whalen JP, Berne AS: The roentgen anatomy of the lateral walls of the orbit (orbital line) and the maxillary antrum (antral line) in the submentovertical view. Am J Roentgenol 91:1009–1011, 1964

Spine

John H. Harris, Jr.

IN DEALING with traumatic lesions of the spine, the radiologist has the opportunity and responsibility to identify the extent and clinical significance of the injury. He therefore plays a major role in the initial management of the patient with an acute spinal injury. Because injuries of the cervical spine are most frequent and have great potential for acute cord damage and delayed instability, the major emphasis in this article will be on cervical spine trauma.

CERVICOCRANIAL INJURIES

The cervicocranium consists of the occiput, the occipitoatlantal joint, the atlas, the axis, and the atlantoaxial articulations. Because of the unique anatomy and physiology of this area and its distinctive response to injury, the cervicocranium is traditionally considered separately from the remainder of the cervical spine.

Anatomic and Physiologic Considerations

Anatomically, it is important to note that the atlas is symmetrically seated on the axis, with the odontoid equidistant from the lateral masses of the atlas, and that the medial and lateral margins of the articulating surfaces of the atlas and the axis are symmetric. The bifid spinous process of C-2 is in the midline (Fig. 1).

The physiologic motions of this area include rotation, lateral bending (gliding, tilt), flexion, extension, and vertical approximation.[9, 12, 13] Vertical approximation refers to the decrease in vertical height of the C-1–C-2 complex that occurs as the biconvex articulating surfaces of the atlas and axis rotate on each other. Flexion and extension occur throughout the cervical area; the least forward and backward displacement occurs at C-7, and displacement becomes progressively greater at each successively higher segment. Normally the interval between the posterior surface of the anterior arch of the atlas and the anterior surface of the dens does not exceed 3 mm in adults[11] in neutral, flexion, and extension positions (Fig. 2). This space is maintained by the tough transverse atlantal ligament (Fig. 3).

Rotation occurs initially as the atlas pivots about the dens. The lateral mass of the atlas, displaced forward during rotation, becomes rectangular in configuration and the space between the lateral mass of the atlas and the dens narrows on that side. The contralateral lateral mass, rotating posteriorly, assumes a truncated configuration, and the dens–lateral mass space is wider (Fig. 4). As rotation increases to maximum degree, the axis rotates in the same direction, resulting in displacement of its bifid spinous process in the opposite direction.

Lateral bending (simple tilting of the head to one side without rotation) results in lateral displacement of the head and atlas (they function as a unit) with respect to the axis (Fig. 5). Thus physiologically the lateral mass of C-1 on the side toward which the head is tilted will be displaced away from the dens, and the dens–lateral mass space on that side will increase in width. On the opposite side, the lateral mass moves toward the dens, and the space is diminished. Early in lateral tilt, the axis rotates in the direction of the tilt, and consequently the spinous process of C-2 rotates off the midline in the opposite direction.

It is necessary to understand these physiologic motions, as demonstrated by Hohl[12, 13] and Fielding,[9] to appreciate the effect that minor imperfections of patient positioning have on the roentgen appearance of the atlantoaxial relationship, to realize that physiologic motions of the cervicocranium may produce radiographic atlantoaxial "offset" and "rotational subluxation," and to understand the roentgen findings in torticollis.

Torticollis

Torticollis is a rotational-tilt deformity of the cervicocranium that typically occurs in childhood and early adolescence. The radiographic findings of torticollis are simply those physio-

John H. Harris, Jr., M.D.: *Chairman, Department of Radiology, Carlisle Hospital, Carlisle, Pa.; Professor of Radiology, Thomas Jefferson University, Philadelphia, Pa.*

Reprint requests should be addressed to Dr. John H. Harris, Jr., Department of Radiology, Carlisle Hospital, 224 Parker St., Carlisle, Pa. 17013.

© *1978 by Grune & Stratton, Inc.*

0037-198X/78/1301-0001/$2.00/0

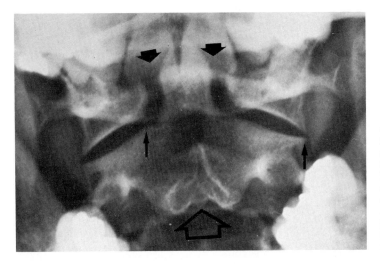

Fig. 1. Open-mouth projection of a normal atlantoaxial articulation. The space between the dens and the lateral masses of the atlas is uniform bilaterally (small arrows), the joint space between the articulating facets is symmetric on the two sides, the medial and lateral margins of the superior and inferior facets are precisely superimposed (small arrows), and the bifid spinous process is in the midline (open arrow).

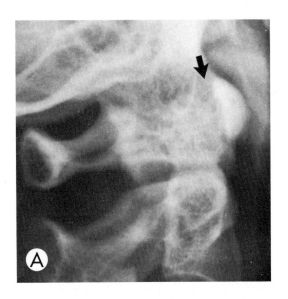

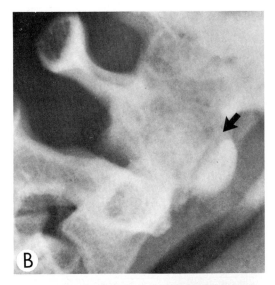

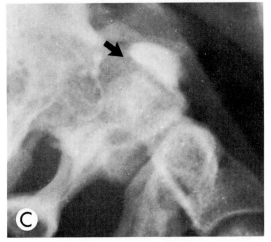

Fig. 2. Lateral radiograph of a normal atlantoaxial articulation in neutral (A), flexion (B), and extension (C) positions. The atlas–dens interval (arrows) does not exceed 3 mm and remains constant in all positions (arrow).

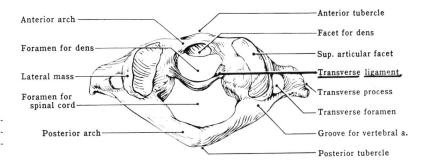

Anterior arch — Anterior tubercle
Foramen for dens — Facet for dens
Lateral mass — Sup. articular facet
Transverse ligament
Foramen for spinal cord — Transverse process
Transverse foramen
Posterior arch — Groove for vertebral a.
Posterior tubercle

Fig. 3. Schematic representation of the atlas, illustrating the transverse atlantal ligament.

logic changes that occur in the atlantoaxial relationship during simultaneous rotation and lateral tilt. These have been described previously. The alterations of the C-1–C-2 relationship of torticollis have been called atlantoaxial rotary displacement by Fielding and Hawkins,[10] and they are illustrated in Figure 6.

Dislocation

Dislocation at the atlanto-occipital level and atlantoaxial rotary dislocation are rarely seen clinically because patients sustaining these injuries usually do not survive.[10]

Fractures of the Dens

Fractures of the odontoid have been classified as type I (avulsion), type II (involving the body),

and type III (basilar)[1] (Fig. 7). Neurologic impairment associated with dens fractures is uncommon and rarely is of major consequence. Type I fractures, which involve the tip of the dens, are uncommon. Type II fractures are the most common. They occur at the junction of the base of the dens and the body of C-2; they are unstable and have the greatest incidence of nonunion. Type III lesions are characterized by the fact that the fracture line extends into the body of the axis. Ninety percent of these fractures unite without incident.

Type II and type III dens fractures may be difficult to identify radiographically. Their detection is facilitated by tomography in frontal and lateral projections (Fig. 8) and by xeroradiography (Fig. 9).

Flexion and extension fractures of the cervicocranial region will be discussed in the next section.

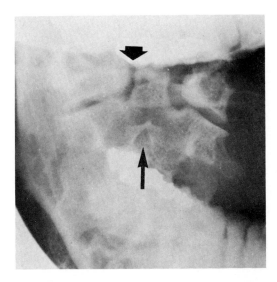

Fig. 4. Frontal view of atlantoaxial articulation with the head rotated moderately to the left in a normal individual. The dens–lateral mass space on the right is narrowed. It is important to realize that even with moderate rotation of the head the axis remains stationary, as shown by the midline position of its spinous process (lower arrow).

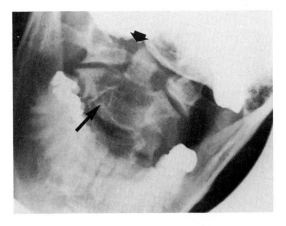

Fig. 5. The atlantoaxial articulation in lateral tilt of the head to the left. The atlas glides laterally to the left, causing the atlantoaxial joints to become asymmetric and the space between the right lateral mass of the atlas and the dens to decrease in width (upper arrow). The axis has rotated to the left, and the spinous process of the axis is displaced from the midline to the right (lower arrow).

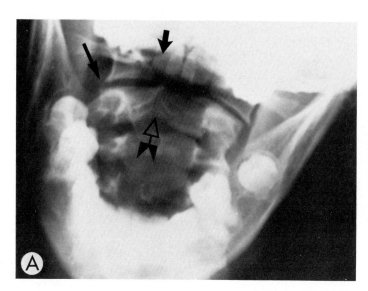
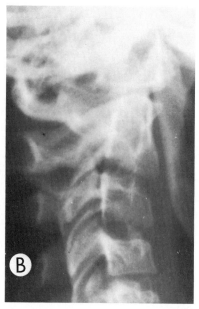

Fig. 6. Atlantoaxial rotary displacement (torticollis, wryneck).(A) Open-mouth projection. The dens is identified through the superimposed maxillary central incisor teeth. The head and atlas are tilted to the left. As a result, the right articular mass of the atlas is medially displaced, decreasing the space between its medial border and the dens (short arrow) and causing the lateral margins of the atlantoaxial articulations to become asymmetric (long arrow). The spinous process of the axis (open arrow) is displaced to the right of the midline, indicating that the axis has rotated in the direction of the tilt (to the left). (B) Lateral projection. The lateral tilt is indicated by loss of definition of the relationship between the anterior arch of C-1 and the dens and by lack of superimposition of the laminae of the posterior arch of the atlas.

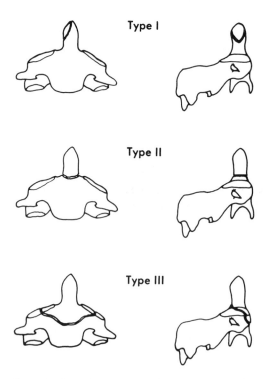

Fig. 7. Classification of odontoid fractures, according to Anderson and D'Alonzo.[1]

OTHER CERVICAL SPINE INJURIES

Understanding the effects of acute cervical spine trauma is enhanced by a pragmatic approach to the mechanisms of injury.[23] Descriptions of the type of cervical injury and its clinical significance are clearer when terms and concepts commonly accepted by orthopedic and neurologic surgeons are used. The concept of acute cervical spine injury that has proved most useful in our practice is based on the work of Holdsworth,[14] Fielding and Hawkins,[10] and Beatson,[3] as modified by personal clinical experience. This concept assumes that each type of lesion is the result of a pure, or dominant mechanism of injury: flexion, flexion-rotation, vertical compression, or extension.

Radiographic Examination

In the severely traumatized patient (one suffering major head or neck injury, multiple organ system injuries or major fractures, unconsciousness, or paralysis), the single most important radiographic examination is the supine, horizontal-beam lateral radiograph of the cer-

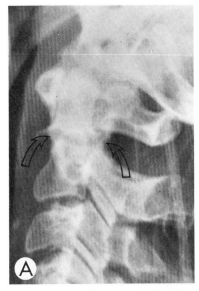

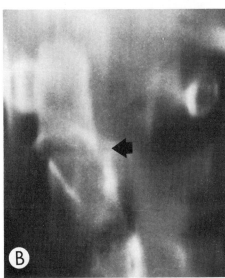

Fig. 8.   Type II fracture of the dens. (A) Routine lateral radiograph. The fracture is not obvious (arrows). (B) Lateral tomograph. The fracture is clearly seen.

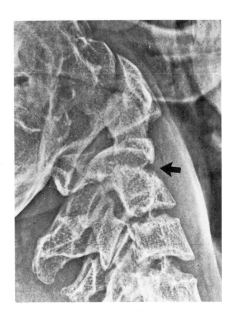

Fig. 9.   Type III fracture of the axis. The fracture was not easily perceived on the lateral radiograph, but it is obvious on this xeroradiograph (arrow). The prevertebral soft-tissue swelling, secondary to hemorrhage, is also well demonstrated by this technique.

diographs indicated. Positioning the patient for these studies should be done under the direct supervision of a physician in order to prevent further cervical cord or nerve root injury from forced flexion or extension.

Acute Cervical Spine Injury

Acute cervical spine injuries are classified according to the mechanism of the trauma (Table 1) and also on the basis of the degree of stability (Table 2). A lesion is considered stable if the patient, initially has no—or minimal—cervical

vical spine. This examination preferably should be made in the emergency room before the patient is moved from the stretcher.

In the less severely injured patient, radiography of the cervical spine should initially be limited to the frontal, lateral, and both oblique projections and should include an "open-mouth" view of the atlantoaxial articulation. Should review of these radiographs be equivocal, or should subluxation be suspected, only then are flexion and extension lateral ra-

Table 1. Mechanisms of Cervical Spine Injuries

Flexion
   Subluxation
   Bilateral interfacetal dislocation
   Simple wedge fracture
   Clay-shoveler's fracture
   Teardrop fracture
Flexion-rotation
   Unilateral interfacetal dislocation
Vertical compression
   Jefferson fracture, C-1
   Burst fracture
Extension
   Posterior neural arch fracture of C-1
   Extension teardrop fracture
   Hangman's fracture

Table 2. Degrees of Stability of Cervical Spine Injuries

Stable
   Subluxation
   Unilateral interfacetal dislocation
   Simple wedge fracture
   Bursting fracture
   Fracture of posterior arch of C-1
Unstable
   Bilateral interfacetal dislocation
   Flexion teardrop fracture
   Extension teardrop fracture
   Hangman's fracture
   Jefferson fracture of C-1

cord or nerve root damage and if cervical spine motion would not be expected to produce cervical cord or nerve root injury. Conversely, an unstable lesion is one in which cervical cord or nerve root injury already exists or in which movement of the cervical spine might produce such injury or aggravate it.

Flexion Injuries

Subluxation

Subluxation consists of minor forward rotation or displacement of one cervical vertebra on

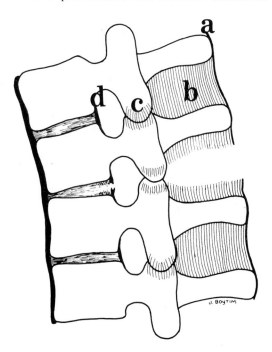

Fig. 10. Schematic representation of subluxation. The posterir ligament complex[14] consists of the supraspinous ligament (a), the interspinous ligament (b), the capsule of the facetal joint (c), and the posterior longitudinal ligament (d). In subluxation, the complex is disrupted, and the posterior portion of the disk is torn.

another. This is accepted as a legitimate entity by orthopedic surgeons,[14,15,23] but it is seldom recognized or accepted by radiologists, despite Cheshire's reported 21% incidence of delayed instability associated with anterior subluxation, as compared to 4%–7% in all types of cervical injury.[7] Delayed instability is defined as the presence of "abnormal mobility between any pair of vertebrae, with or without pain or other clinical manifestation, when lateral x-rays of the cervical spine are taken in flexion and extension at the conclusion of conservative treatment."[7]

Subluxation is the result of a purely soft-tissue injury consisting of disruption of the posterior ligament complex (the supraspinous, interspinous, and posterior longitudinal ligaments, the capsule of the interfacetal joints, and the ligamentum flavum) and, in addition, a tear of the posterior portion of the intervertebral disk (Fig. 10).[14]

Radiographically, in the neutral lateral projection the interspinous space *is* widened at the level of subluxation. This has been referred to as *fanning* by Fielding and Hawkins.[10] The superior facets are displaced upward and forward with respect to the contiguous inferior facets of the joint. The disk space is widened posteriorly and narrowed anteriorly as a result of rotation of the involved vertebral body on its anterior inferior corner. These signs are aggravated in flexion and are reduced in extension (Fig. 11). Delayed instability 1 year after acute subluxation of C-3 on C-4 is illustrated in Fig. 12.

Bilateral Interfacetal Dislocation

Bilateral interfacetal dislocation (BID) is considered by most authors to be the result of straight forced flexion. It is characterized by complete disruption of the posterior ligament complex, the posterior longitudinal ligament, the annulus, and frequently the anterior longitudinal ligament[3], and by complete anterior dislocation of the superior facets with respect to the inferior facets of the involved joints. The dislocated facets pass upward and forward over the inferior facets of the joint and come to rest in the intervertebral foramina.

With complete BID, the superior facets are seen radiographically to lie fully anterior to the inferior facets. The body of the dislocated segment is displaced anteriorly a distance greater

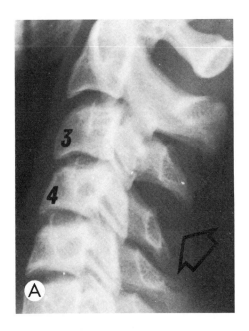

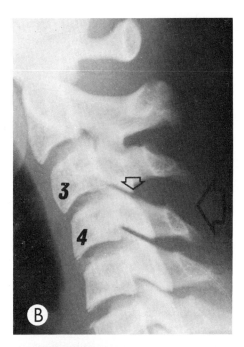

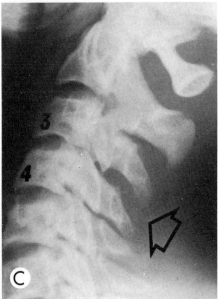

Fig. 11. Subluxation of C-3 and C-4. (A) In the neutral lateral projection, the third vertebra is rotated anteriorly, resulting in discontinuity of the normal cervical lordotic curve at the level of the third interspace. The disk space is narrowed anteriorly and widened posteriorly. The interspinous space is abnormally widened (arrow). (B) In flexion, all of the changes seen in (A) are exaggerated. The superior facets of the facetal joints at C-3–C-4 are displaced anteriorly with respect to the inferior facets, as indicated by the positions of their posterior inferior margins (small arrow). There is further widening of the C-3–C-4 interspinous space (large arrow). (C) In extension, all of the changes recorded in (A) and (B) are reversed, and the spine assumes a normal appearance.

than one-half of the AP diameter of the body below. This amount of forward displacement, as seen in the lateral radiograph of the cervical spine, is indicative of BID. Beatson,[3] using human cadaveric cervical spine specimens, demonstrated that it is impossible to produce BID without this degree of forward displacement of the vertebral body. When this characteristic radiographic picture is seen on the horizontal-beam lateral radiograph, additional

studies are contraindicated because of the gross instability of BID.

When the dislocation is not complete, oblique views (personally supervised by the radiologist) may be required to establish the bilaterality of the lesion (Fig. 13).

BID is associated with a high incidence of cord damage, and because of the skeletal dislocation and the disruption of all the soft-tissue structures, it is mechanically unstable. BID is

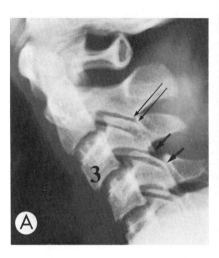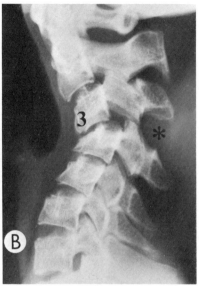

Fig. 12. Delayed instability. (A) Subluxation of C-3 on C-4. The body of C-3 is displaced anteriorly. The long arrows indicate the posterior margins of one facetal joint at the C-2–C-3 level. The short arrows indicate the abnormal relationships of the posterior margins of the facets at the level of subluxation. (B) The same patient 11 months after injury. The C-3–C-4 relationship reflects further displacement of C-3 and evidence of delayed instability. The interspinous space (asterisk) is wider than in A.

invariably associated with a tiny (usually insignificant) fracture that arises from the margin of one of the dislocated facets.[4]

Wedge Fracture

The simple wedge fracture (Fig. 14) consists of anterior compression of the involved vertebral body between the adjacent vertebral bodies. The injury is stable and, alone, is rarely accompanied by central nervous system signs.

Clay-shoveler's Fracture

The clay-shoveler's fracture (Fig. 15) is an oblique fracture of the base of the spinous process of one of the lower cervical segments, usually C-7. The injury derives its name from its common occurrence in clay miners in Australia during the 1930s. In this injury, abrupt flexion of the head, in opposition to the force of the supraspinous ligament, results in fracture of the spinous process. Since the fracture involves only the spinous process, the lesion is stable and is not associated with neurologic damage.

Flexion Teardrop Fracture

The flexion teardrop fracture-dislocation[20] is the most severe and the most unstable injury of the cervical spine. The lesion is characterized radiographically by forward dislocation of the involved vertebra, fracture or dislocation of its

posterior elements, and complete disruption of all the soft tissues at the level of injury (Fig. 16). The lesion is therefore totally unstable and is associated with the *acute anterior cervical cord syndrome,* which is defined as immediate complete motor paralysis and loss of anterior column sensations (pain and temperature), but retention of the posterior column senses of position, vibration, and motion.[19]

A few authors[3,14,18] have considered the flexion teardrop fracture and the *burst fracture* (caused by vertical compression) to be the same entity; however, the majority have recognized that their mechanisms of injury and pathophysiology differ, that their roentgen appearances, while sometimes similar, are distinctive, and that there is a significant difference between their neurologic complications. Because of these distinguishing characteristics, the flexion teardrop fracture and the burst fracture are considered to be distinct injuries.

Flexion-Rotation Injury

Unilateral Interfacetal Fracture

Unilateral interfacetal dislocation is the only injury of the cervical spine caused by a flexion-rotation mechanism. The rotational component occurs about one of the interfacetal joints, which acts as the fulcrum. Simultaneous flexion and rotation cause the contralateral interfacetal joint to dislocate, with the superior facet riding

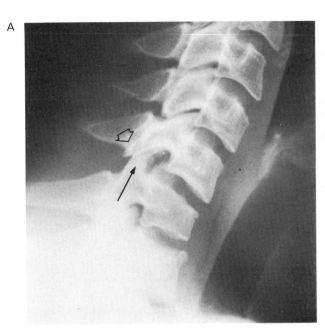

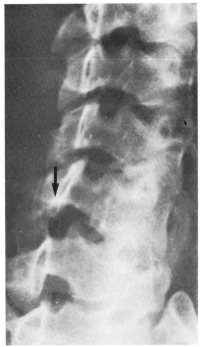

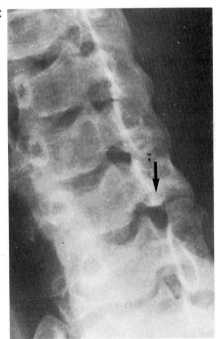

Fig. 13. Incomplete bilateral interfacetal dislocation of C-6 on C-7. (A) The solid arrow indicates the position of each superior facet of the joint anterior to the inferior facets. The open arrow designates a small clinically insignificant fracture at the side of dislocation. Simple wedge fractures involve the bodies of C-7 and T-1. (B and C) The oblique projections confirm the dislocation of the superior facet of each facetal joint at the involved level (arrows).

upward, forward, and over the tip of the inferior facet and coming to rest within the intervertebral foramen anterior to the subjacent articular mass. In this position, the dislocated articular mass is mechanically locked or perched in place. Unilateral interfacetal dislocation is mechanically stable,[5] even though the posterior ligament complex is disrupted.

Because of the rotational component of unilateral interfacetal dislocation, the frontal projection of the cervical spine demonstrates that the spinous processes from the level of disloca-

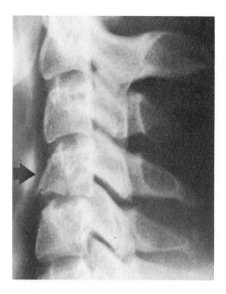

Fig. 14. Simple wedge fracture of C-4 (arrow).

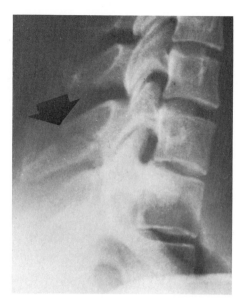

Fig. 15. Clay-shoveler's fracture (arrow).

tion upward are displaced from the midline in the direction of the rotation. In the lateral radiograph the lesion is characterized by forward displacement of the dislocated segment on the vertebra below and by rotation of the dislocated vertebra and those above it. Oblique projections are required to identify the dislocated facetal joint, which is fundamental to successful management of this lesion (Fig. 17).

Vertical Compression

Vertical compression injuries occur only in those segments of the spine that are capable of

voluntary straightening (the cervical and lumbar region). Compression injuries in the cervical spine include the Jefferson fracture of the atlas and the burst (bursting, compression, or dispersion) fracture that occurs in the middle or lower cervical segments. These fractures are caused by the transmittal of force through the spine either from above downward (through the skull) or from below upward (through the pelvis). They are uncommon, because the impact must occur at the precise instant that the normal cervical lordotic curve is straightened.

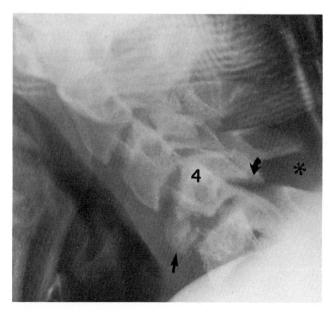

Fig. 16. Flexion teardrop fracture of C-4. This teenage boy dove from a height into a shallow stream, sustaining the fracture illustrated. He was instantly paralyzed from the neck down, and he remains so 10 years later. The upper cervical segments are angulated anteriorly, indicating a flexion type of injury. The anterior inferior corner fragment (lower arrow) is separated from the remainder of the vertebra. These two characteristics are the basis for the name *flexion teardrop*. The intervertebral disk is disrupted. The position of the separate anterior fragment and the position of the posterior inferior corner of the body indicate that the anterior and posterior longitudinal ligaments are disrupted. The abnormal relationship of the interfacetal joints (upper arrow) and the fanning (asterisk) indicate that the posterior ligament complex is torn.

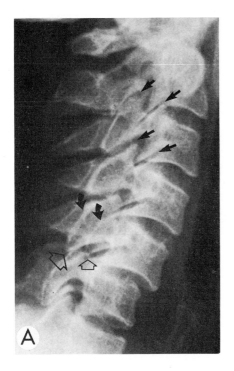

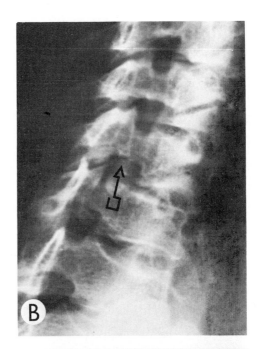

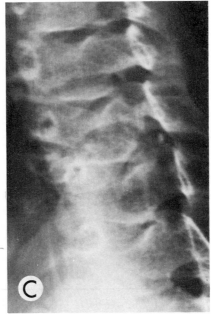

Fig. 17. Unilateral interfacetal dislocation. (A) In the neutral lateral radiograph, anterior dislocation of C-5 is obvious. The dislocated superior facet lies anterior to its contiguous inferior facet (right open arrow). The opposite interfacetal joint at the same level shows the superior facet normally seated posterior to the inferior facet (left open arrow). The rotational component is manifested by the fact that the posterior cortex of the articular mass on the dislocated side lies anterior to its mate (curved arrows), as does the interfacetal joint space (straight arrows). (B) Right oblique projection. The dislocated facet (arrow) lies within the intervertebral foramen. (C) No dislocation exists on the opposite side in the left oblique view.

Jefferson Fracture

The Jefferson fracture of C-1 was first described in 1920,[16] and by 1970 only 191 cases had been reported in the world literature.[22] Classically, it is the result of symmetric transmittal of force through the occipital condyles to the superior articular surfaces of the lateral masses of the atlas. This drives the lateral masses laterally, resulting in fractures of each side of the anterior and posterior arches of the atlas, as well as disruption of the transverse atlantal ligament. In the typical form of the injury, the lateral displacements of the two articular masses are equal. Atypically, the force may be applied eccentrically to the skull and transmitted to one of the lateral masses of the

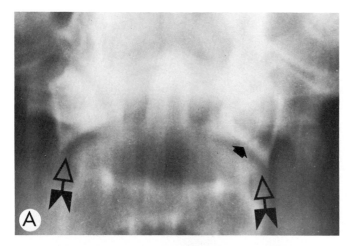

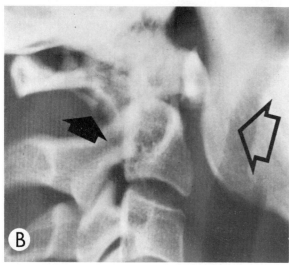

Fig. 18. Jefferson fracture of the atlas, frontal tomogram. (A) The lateral masses of the atlas are uniformly displaced with respect to the dens and the lateral margins of the superior facets of the axis (open arrows). The fracture of the left lateral mass (solid arrow) was not recognizable on plain radiographs. (B) In the lateral view a prevertebral soft-tissue mass, representing hemorrhage, is seen (open arrow). The minimally displaced fragments of the posterior arch of C-1 are indicated by the solid arrow.

atlas in greater magnitude than to the other. In that instance, displacement of the articular pillars will be asymmetric.

When the fragments are minimally displaced, the Jefferson fracture is difficult to recognize radiographically. In the frontal projection, because of the lateral displacement of the lateral masses of the atlas, the atlas-dens interval is symmetrically widened, and the lateral margins of the inferior articulating facets of the atlas lie lateral to the margins of the superior facets of the axis (Fig. 18). In a lateral radiograph, there is often a soft-tissue mass produced by the accompanying prevertebral hemorrhage. The space between the posterior surface of the anterior ring of the atlas and the anterior surface of the dens widens to exceed 3mm, and fragments of the bilateral fractures involving the superimposed laminae may be visible. Tomog-

raphy in both frontal and lateral projections may be necessary to demonstrate the Jefferson fracture.

Burst Fracture

The burst fracture results when the nucleus pulposus is driven through the endplate into the vertebral body at the instant of impact, fracturing the vertebra vertically. Further intrusion of the nucleus into the vertebra causes the body to explode from within, resulting in comminution.[2,17] Typically the posterior inferior fragment is posteriorly displaced and may impinge upon or penetrate the ventral surface of the cord. Although this lesion may be associated with paraplegia, the frequency and magnitude of neurologic damage are much less than those that occur with the flexion teardrop fracture.

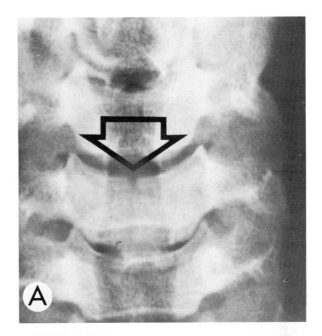

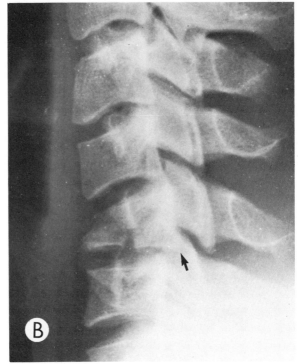

Fig. 19. Burst fracture. (A) The characteristic vertical fracture of the vertebral body (arrow) is seen in the frontal view. (B) In the lateral radiograph, the general alignment of the cervical vertebrae is in the military position, characteristic of the burst fracture. The involved body is comminuted, with the posterior inferior fragment driven posteriorly to encroach on the spinal canal (arrow). The interfacetal joints and the majority of the posterior ligament complex remain intact. Compare this lesion with the flexion teardrop fracture (Fig. 7).

The burst fracture is considered to be stable, because the anterior longitudinal ligament, the capsule of the facetal joints, and the interspinous and supraspinous ligaments are all intact, and because the integrity of the facetal joints is maintained.

The frontal radiograph demonstrates the characteristic vertical fracture of the vertebral body, which helps differentiate the burst fracture from the simple wedge fracture and the flexion teardrop fracture. In the lateral projection, the vertebral body is comminuted, and typically, the posterior inferior fragment is displaced posteriorly into the spinal canal (Fig. 19).

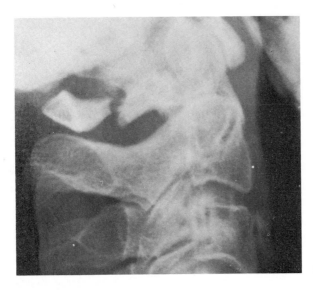

Fig. 20.   Fracture of the posterior arch of the atlas.

Extension Injuries

Posterior Neural Arch Fracture of C-1

The simplest of the extension fractures involves the posterior ring of the atlas (Fig. 20) and results from compression of the posterior elements between the occiput and the heavy spinous process of the axis. The fracture is stable because the anterior ring and the transverse atlantal ligament are intact.

Extension Teardrop Fracture

The extension teardrop fracture typically involves the axis. The anterior longitudinal ligament is attached to the anterior inferior corner of the axis. During forced abrupt extension, the dense, tough anterior longitudinal ligament may pull the anterior inferior corner of the axis away from the remainder of the vertebral body, producing the classic triangular-shaped fracture (Fig. 21). This fracture is stable in flexion but unstable in extension.

Hangman's Fracture

The hangman's fracture (traumatic spondylolisthesis) occurs when the cervicocranium (the skull, atlas, and axis functioning as a unit) is

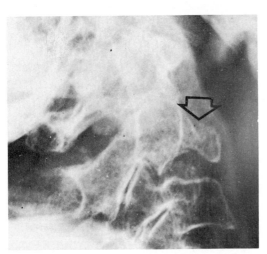

Fig. 21.   Extension teardrop fracture.

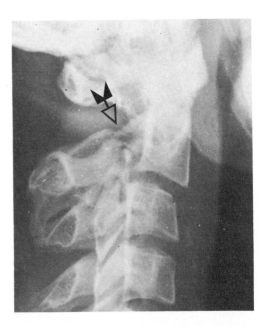

Fig. 22.   Hangman's fracture of the axis. The body of the axis is anteriorly displaced. Bilateral pedicle fractures are present (arrow). Anterior prevertebral soft-tissue swelling reflects the presence of retropharyngeal hemorrhage.

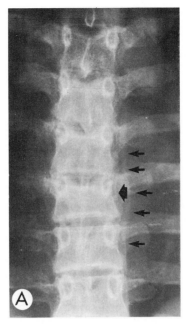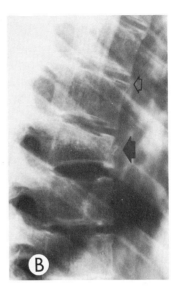

Fig. 23. Vertebral fracture. (A) In the frontal projection, bulging of the mediastinal stripe (small arrows) signals the presence of a subtle acute fracture of the vertebral body (large arrow). (B) In the lateral radiograph, the fracture is indicated by the solid arrow. The open arrow indicates an ununited ring epiphysis.

thrown into extreme hyperextension as a result of abrupt deceleration from high speed.[8,21] This injury is more commonly the result of a head-on automobile accident than the result of hanging. There is bilateral fracture of the pedicles of the axis, with or without associated dislocation (Fig. 22). Although the lesion is unstable, cord damage is usually minimal because the AP diameter of the neural canal is greatest at the C-2 level and because the bilateral pedicle fractures permit the spinal canal to decompress itself.

THORACIC SPINE

Fractures of the thoracic spine usually do not pose diagnostic problems. However, three points relative to thoracic spine injuries do merit recitation:

1. The upper three or four thoracic vertebrae are generally not seen on the routine lateral radiograph of either the cervical or thoracic spine. Tomography and "off-lateral" radiographs made in the Fletcher position are required for adequate evaluation of the upper thoracic segments.

2. Localized bulging of the mediastinal stripe (Fig. 23) may be the only roentgenologic evidence of a subtle thoracic vertebral body fracture. But, of course, this sign may also be produced by infection or neoplasm.

3. Multiple or severe fractures of the upper thoracic vertebrae may cause posterior mediastinal hemorrhage of sufficient magnitude to produce ill-defined mediastinal widening similar to that attributed to traumatic rupture of the aorta. In these instances, emergency aortography is essential to establish that the aorta is intact. Horizontal-beam lateral radiographs of the thoracic spine will usually es-

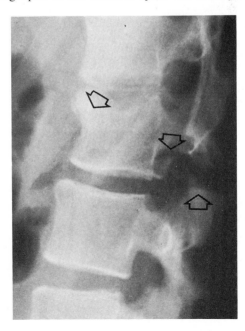

Fig. 24. Chance fracture (arrows).

tablish the presence and magnitude of the vertebral fractures.

LUMBAR SPINE INJURIES

Fractures of the lumbar transverse processes are common and are easily overlooked. Hemorrhage contained within the psoas muscle often causes bulging of its lateral margin. Displacement of the fragments is often associated with severe tearing of the psoas muscle, frank retro-

peritoneal hemorrhage, and obliteration of the psoas shadow. Fractures of the transverse processes of L-2 and L-3 should lead one to consider renal trauma.

The Chance fracture[6] is a lumbar spine fracture that results from a shearing flexion mechanism. It is an obliquely horizontal fracture of the spinous process and neural arch, extending through the superior portion of the vertebral body (Fig. 24).

REFERENCES

1. Anderson LD, D'Alonzo RT: Fractures of the odontoid process of the axis. J Bone Joint Surg 56A: 1663–1691, 1974

2. Apley AG: Fractures of the spine. Ann R Coll Surg Engl 46: 210–223, 1970

3. Beatson TR: Fractures and dislocations of the cervical spine. J Bone Joint Surg 45B: 21–35, 1963

4. Bedbrook GM. Stability of spinal fractures and fracture dislocations. Paraplegia 9:23–32, 1971

5. Braakman R, Vinken PJ: Unilateral facet interlocking in the lower cervical spine. J Bone Joint Surg 49B: 249–257, 1967

6. Chance GQ: Note on type of flexion fracture of spine. Br J Radiol 21: 452–453, 1948

7. Cheshire DJ: The stability of the cervical spine following the conservative treatment of fractures and fracture-dislocations. Paraplegia 7:193–203, 1969

8. Cornish BL: Traumatic spondylolisthesis of the axis. J Bone Joint Surg 50B: 31–43, 1968

9. Fielding JW: Cineroentgenography of the normal cervical spine. J Bone Joint Surg 39A: 1280–1288, 1957

10. Fielding JW, Hawkins RJ: Roentgenographic Diagnosis of the Injured Neck, Chapter 7, p 149. Instructional course lectures, American Academy of Orthopedic Surgeons, vol 25. St. Louis, CV Mosby, 1976

11. Hinck VC, Hopkins CE: Measurement of the atlanto-dental interval in the adult. Am J Roentgenol 84:945–951, 1960

12. Hohl M: Normal motions in the upper portion of the cervical spine. J Bone Joint Surg 46A: 1777–1779, 1964

13. Hohl M, Baker HR: The atlanto-axial joint. Roentgenographic and anatomic study of normal and abnormal motion. J Bone Joint Surg 46:1739–1752, 1964

14. Holdsworth F: Fractures, dislocations and fracture-dislocations of the spine. J Bone Joint Surg 52A: 1534–1551, 1970

15. Jackson R: Updating the neck. Trauma 1:7–89, 1970

16. Jefferson G: Fracture of the atlas vertebra. Report of four cases and a review of those previously recorded. Br J Surg 7:407–422, 1920

17. Roaf R: A study of the mechanics of spinal injuries. J Bone Joint Surg 42B:810–823, 1960

18. Rothman RH, Simeone FA (eds): The Spine. Philadelphia, WB Saunders, 1975

19. Schneider RC: Chronic neurological sequelae of acute trauma to the spine and spinal cord. Part V. The syndrome of acute central cervical spinal cord injury followed by chronic anterior cervical cord injury (or compression) syndrome. J Bone Joint Surg 42A: 253–260, 1960

20. Schneider RC, Kahn EA: Chronic neurological sequelae of acute trauma to the spine and spinal cord. Part I. The significance of the acute-flexion or "tear-drop" fracture-dislocation of the cervical spine. J Bone Joint Surg 38A: 985–997, 1956

21. Schneider RC, Livingston KE, Cave AJ, et al.: "Hangman's fracture" of the cervical spine. J Neurosurg 22: 141–154, 1965

22. Sherk K, Nicholson JT: Fractures of the atlas. J Bone Joint Surg 52A: 1017–1024, 1970

23. Stringa G: Traumatic lesions of the cervical spine—statistics, mechanism, classification, in: Proceedings of the IXth Congress of the International Society of Orthopaedic Surgery and Traumatology. Brussels, Imprimerie des Sciences, pp 69-97, 1963

Bony Thorax

Kenneth R. Kattan

THE automobile accident is the single greatest cause of closed chest injury, and it carries the highest mortality rate.[14] Although the bony thorax and the shoulder girdle offer partial protection to the thoracic viscera, they are ineffective against a penetrating injury or the sudden deceleration experienced in an automobile collision. A patient who has sustained rib fractures should be examined for possible injury to the pleura, lungs, or blood vessels, while the thoracic cage itself takes a secondary place in management. In the occasional patient who breaks a rib or two during a severe coughing episode, injury to internal structures is minimal.

Fracture of the upper three ribs may signal more serious injury to the tracheobronchial tree and the vascular structures.[4,6,23] Injury to the lower three ribs may be associated with laceration of the liver, spleen, or kidney. In childhood, the ribs are resilient, but they become more rigid and brittle with advancing age, so that the incidence of rib fracture increases after the third decade.[24] Pathologic fractures and trauma resulting from penetrating injuries will not be discussed here because of space limitation.

TRAUMA OF THE RIB CAGE

Trauma of the thoracic cage most commonly involves the fourth through the ninth ribs (Figs. 1 and 2). The shoulder girdle and muscles form a protective buffer for the upper three ribs (Fig. 3). The lower three ribs, being more mobile and more yielding than the true ribs, are broken less frequently.

The number of ribs affected and the degree of displacement depend on the type and severity of the injury. If force is applied in an AP direction over a wide area, the ribs may buckle outward, resulting in fracture of several ribs without injury to the underlying viscera.

Fractures of the costal cartilage are more painful and less common than fractures of the osseous part. Cartilage fractures are difficult to demonstrate radiologically. Fracture of the sternum may be accompanied by costal cartilage fracture.[14]

The severely crushed chest warrants special attention. This type of injury usually causes segmental fractures of several ribs, accompanied by separation at their costochondral junctions or by fracture of the sternum. Consequently, the section of fractured ribs loses continuity with the rest of the thoracic wall, thus becoming "flail." The flail segment moves in the opposite direction from the rest of the thoracic cage during respiration (Fig. 4). During inspiration, these separate flail segments move inward; during expiration they move outward. Ventilatory efficiency is reduced if the flail segment involves a large number of ribs. Impaired ventilation is present in the normal lung because of partial passage of air from the injured lung to the normal lung during inspiration and passage in the opposite direction during expiration. This has been called *pendulum breathing*. Cough becomes ineffective, and secretions are retained in the bronchial tree. There is reduction of gaseous exchange. These factors result in hypoxia and pulmonary edema, leading to traumatic wet lung syndrome.[14]

Many publications have given the impression that radiologic examination is unreliable in the diagnosis of rib fractures. This impression is true if the diagnosis is reached on the basis of only a single film of the chest.[13] Bavendam and Nedelman[1] reported a case in which one rib fracture was seen on the first day, with follow-up films showing four fractures, then six fractures; after 4 weeks callus was seen in eight fractured ribs.

The commonly used projections are the following:[19]

1. The AP (or PA) film; this adequately shows the anterior and posterior thirds of the ribs

Kenneth R. Kattan, M.D.: *Radiology Service, Veterans Administration Center; Professor and Vice-Chairman, Department of Radiological Sciences, Wright State University School of Medicine, Dayton, Ohio.*

Reprint requests should be addressed to Kenneth R. Kattan, M.D., Department of Radiology, Veterans Administration Hospital, 4100 West Third Street, Dayton, Ohio.

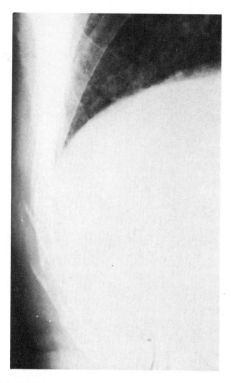

Fig. 1. Fracture of the axillary portion of the eighth and ninth right ribs. The displacement and location enable us to recognize the fracture in this section of a PA teleroentgenogram of the chest. Incidental finding on a routine chest film of a 66-year-old white man with hemorrhoids.

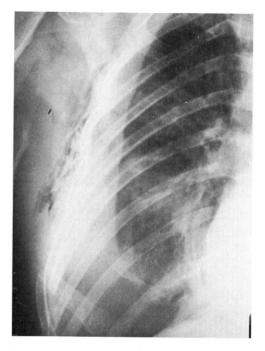

Fig. 2. Fracture of fifth to eighth right ribs on an AP recumbent roentgenogram. Chest wall emphysema is noted, as are large amounts of air and fluid in the pleural cavity. Note that the diaphragm is well delineated with air density and an absence of bronchovascular markings in the base of the right hemithorax.

above the diaphragm. The upright position is preferable because in this position the diaphragm takes a lower position and therefore more ribs are shown.

2. A well-penetrated AP film for the lower ribs, below the diaphragm.
3. Oblique views for the axillary part of the ribs.
4. Coned views over areas of suspected fracture.

It is essential, in the severely injured patient, first to maintain an open airway, control hemorrhage, and reverse shock.[7,14] In these patients, only a recumbent chest film can be obtained, and therefore a slight degree of hemothorax or pneumothorax may be missed. In the supine position, fluid accumulates in the posterior part of the pleural cavity, giving a uniform increase in density without obliteration of the bronchovascular markings.[10] A smaller amount of fluid may be manifested by widening of the posterior mediastinal stripe.[27] A decubitus film

is more useful than a supine film, since it detects smaller amounts of fluid and also shows shifting of the density if the fluid is not loculated. It is well known that an expiration film is helpful in demonstrating a small pneumothorax.

The fracture is easily recognized on a properly exposed film when the fracture line is more or less perpendicular to the x-ray beam. On the other hand, it is difficult to recognize the fracture line when it is parallel to the beam unless the fragments are displaced. Local extrapleural hematoma is a useful indirect sign of fracture when the fracture itself is not seen. It resembles pleural thickening (Fig. 3B).

INJURY TO THE PLEURA

Injury to the pleura is recognized by hemothorax (Fig. 2) or pneumothorax. The technical factors used in the radiographic study of the ribs are apt to obscure a pneumothorax (Fig. 3A). If possible, the patient should be placed in the upright position, and an expiratory chest film should be obtained to enhance pneumothorax. A

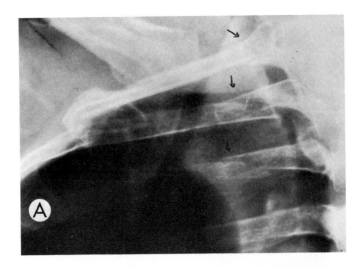

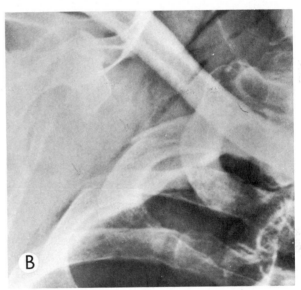

Fig. 3. Fracture of the posterior parts of the first, second, and third right ribs (arrows). This 60-year-old white man fell while fishing. He was dyspneic on admission. (A) In this right posterior oblique position, the ribs are parallel to the table. Pneumothorax is present, but it cannot be recognized in this overexposed film. (B) Right anterior oblique position. The fractures of the second and third ribs are seen and show slight displacement. Note the localized extrapleural shadow caused by the hematoma, as well as soft-tissue emphysema.

false impression of pneumothorax may be caused by linear shadows of clothes, bedsheets, or skin folds. These shadows are linear and do not conform to the curvilinear edge of the collapsed lung, which is nearly parallel to the chest wall. The shadows produced by subcutaneous emphysema may obscure a pneumothorax.

Hemothorax is caused by injury to the blood vessels in the chest wall, lung, diaphragm, or mediastinum. Blood accumulating in the pleural cavity from the lung tends to compress the pulmonary blood vessels, so that the tamponade effect reduces the bleeding. This is not the case in hemothorax of other origin.[24,29]

INJURY TO LUNG PARENCHYMA

Pulmonary contusion is the most common lesion caused by nonpenetrating injury to the chest, even more frequent than rib fractures.[28] Roentgenographically, it appears within 6 hr after injury as a dense, irregular, patchy area of alveolar infiltrate. This opacity seldom conforms to a segment or lobe of the lung (Fig. 5). Improvement is seen within 48 hr, with complete resolution within 3–10 days. If progressive clearing has not occurred by 72 hr after the trauma, pulmonary laceration, pneumonia, or atelectasis should be suspected.[8,26]

Penetrating injuries are the usual causes of

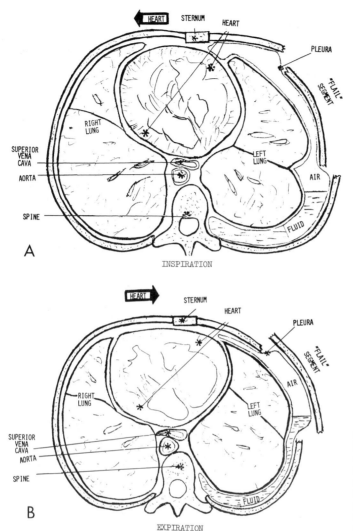

Fig. 4. Diagrammatic cross section of the motion in flail chest. (A) Inspiration. (B) Expiration. The separate segment of rib sinks inward during inspiration and bulges outward during expiration. The mediastinum moves toward the normal side during inspiration. There is also movement of air from the injured lung to the normal lung during inspiration and the reverse during expiration.

pulmonary hematoma or laceration, but these can also follow severe blunt trauma. A pulmonary hematoma is a laceration that has filled with blood.[29] Initially, the shadow of the hematoma is usually obscured by that of the surrounding contusion. As the contusion clears, a circular or elliptic area filled with air and/or blood appears (Fig. 6). If it is filled with blood only, air may appear later as a crescent at the periphery of the clot. Later still, the crescent of air disappears, and a circular density remains. In the absence of a history or previous films for comparison, this density may be mistaken for a neoplasm (Fig. 6B).

SPLENIC RUPTURE

Although the spleen is relatively well protected by the ribs posteriorly and laterally and is cushioned by the surrounding organs anteriorly, it is one of the most frequently injured organs following nonpenetrating trauma of the trunk.[25] Fractured left ribs commonly accompany splenic rupture, but splenic injury frequently occurs without rib fractures. Early diagnosis and surgery are prerequisite for survival.

Plain films of the abdomen show a soft-tissue shadow in the splenic area, larger than the normal spleen (Fig. 7). Displacement to the right, indentation on the stomach, and downward displacement of the splenic flexure are significant signs.[12] Collection of fluid in the left paracolic gutter is an additional sign. Elevation of the left hemidiaphragm, left-sided pleural effusion, and gastric dilatation are nonspecific secondary signs of splenic injury.

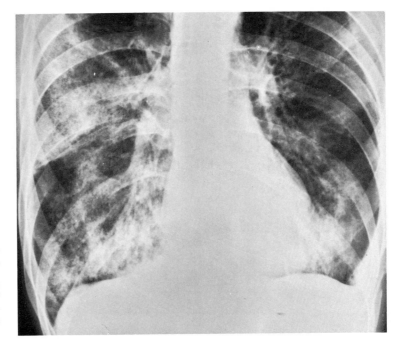

Fig. 5. Pulmonary contusion several hours after a deceleration injury. Fracture of the eighth and ninth left ribs has occurred with slight bleeding into the overlying extrapleural space. There are multiple areas of alveolar infiltrate in the lower and middle lung fields bilaterally. Eleven days later the lung fields were clear.

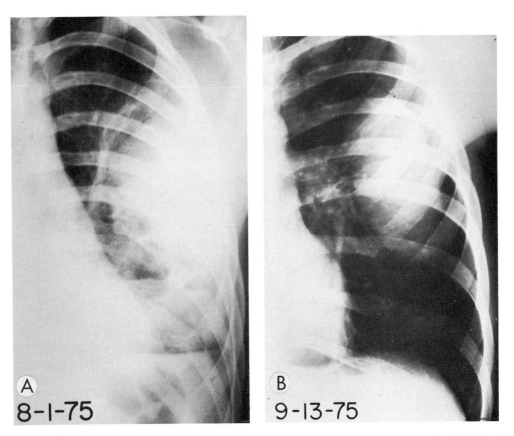

Fig. 6. Pulmonary laceration with hematoma. (A) Several days after a tractor injury; note the multiple air-fluid levels in the large density. (B) Six weeks later; the hematoma has organized into a large, well-defined homogeneous density. (Courtesy of Drs. Jerome F. Wiot and John A. Parlin, Cincinnati, Ohio.)

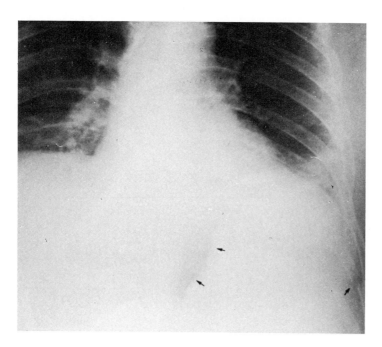

Angiography and radioisotope scans of the spleen are helpful tools in the diagnosis. Scanning is less accurate and less specific than angiography. An ultrasound scan will show the extravasated blood as a sonolucent area and will show enlargement of the spleen. The tear in the spleen is difficult to recognize.[11] The possibility of delayed hemorrhage should be considered. The latent period before frank rupture takes place may be from 48 hr to several days.[25]

INJURY TO TRACHEOBRONCHIAL TREE

Tracheobronchial injury is caused by severe compression of the AP diameter of the chest. The overall mortality is 30%, with 50% dying in the first hour.[9] Pneumothorax, pneumomediastinum, and chest wall emphysema are the usual findings. Another frequent complication of this injury is atelectasis of a lobe or an entire lung. Failure of the atelectatic lung to reexpand after

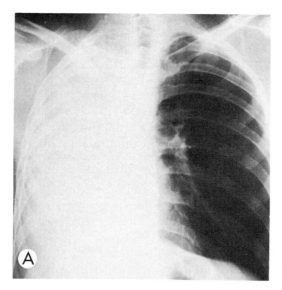
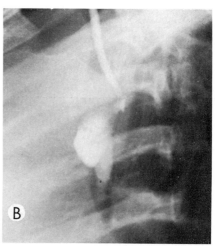

Fig. 8. Injury to the right main bronchus with collapse of the right lung in an automobile accident. (A) The displacement of the mediastinum to the right is striking. Fractures of the right clavicle and the second rib anteriorly are present. (B) Bronchogram showing a block of the right main bronchus. (Courtesy of Dr. Charles F. Mueller, Columbus, Ohio.)

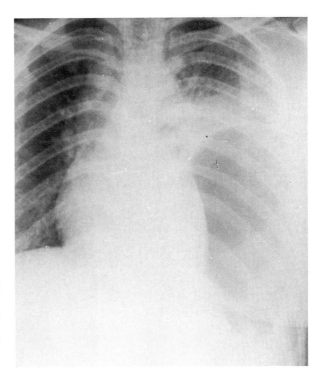

Fig. 9. Rupture of left hemidiaphragm. The shadow of the distended stomach in the left chest resembles an elevated left hemidiaphragm. This 30-year-old woman was admitted after an accident with tenderness of the seventh, eighth, and ninth ribs in the midaxillary line. On a film 1 day earlier, fractures of the ninth and tenth ribs were seen, and the stomach was in normal position. At operation, two tears were found in the diaphragm. The stomach was in the left hemithorax. There was also contusion of the pancreas.

the introduction of a chest tube for pneumothorax is suggestive of bronchial rupture. Fracture of the first or second rib should also raise the possibility of injury to the trachea or the main bronchi (Fig. 8). A specific sign of complete bronchial rupture is shift of the collapsed lung to the most dependent part of the thorax with change in the patient's position.

If atelectasis does not appear immediately after bronchial trauma, it may be seen later if bronchial stenosis develops. This occurs within 2 months after the trauma.[6] High kilovoltage roentgenograms and tomography can aid in the discovery of bronchial narrowing before the advent of atelectasis. Bronchography is rarely necessary.[4]

INJURY TO DIAPHRAGM

The incidence of diaphragmatic injury has risen as a consequence of the increase in traffic accidents. Compression of the chest or abdomen, particularly by the steering wheel, is the most common cause of diaphragmatic rupture.[16] The left side is affected in 95% of cases because the right hemidiaphragm is protected by the liver.[16] In 90% of cases the diagnosis is missed in the early posttraumatic period.[2]

Trauma of sufficient severity to cause injury to the diaphragm will frequently injure other structures[21] (Fig. 9). In a review of 261 patients with traumatic diaphragmatic hernia, Hood found a 78% incidence of rib or other skeletal fracture.[17] Splenic rupture was present in 35% and hepatic rupture in 6% of the same series.

The roentgenographic findings may be summarized as follows: (1) abnormally high "hemidiaphragm"; (2) gas shadows above the normal level of the diaphragm; (3) shift of the mediastinal shadows to the contralateral side; (4) diskoid atelectasis at the lung base.[5] Bleeding in the pleural cavity is a nonspecific sign of diaphragmatic rupture.

Filling of the stomach or colon with contrast medium will verify the hernia and recognition of obstruction, incarceration, or strangulation. These latter complications may appear several years after the accident.[3, 10]

Right-sided diaphragmatic hernia may also give the impression of an elevated hemidiaphragm if the tear is large and much or all of the liver moves into the chest.[22] If the tear is small, a small portion of liver may mushroom through the tear. The radioisotope liver scan will show that what appears to be a lung tumor is in fact liver tissue. The diagnosis is obvious in

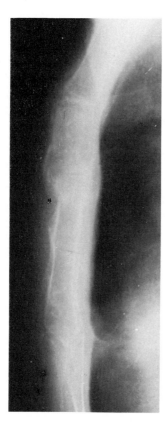

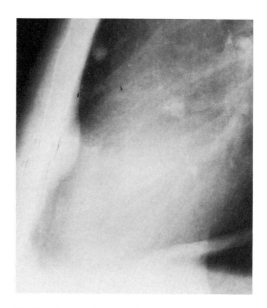

Fig. 11.   Recent fracture of the sternum. Note the extra-pleural shadow due to hematoma at the site of the fracture (retouched).

Fig. 10.   Fracture of the sternum with displacement. This 79-year-old patient had fallen 9 days previously.

the few instances in which bowel herniates through the right hemidiaphragm.

FRACTURE OF STERNUM

Injury to the sternum is in most cases caused by direct trauma. It may result in dislocation at the manubriosternal synchondrosis or fracture through the body of the sternum. In most cases the fracture is transverse and the displacement is slight (Fig. 10). A localized soft-tissue swelling behind or in front of the sternum is usually seen when the trauma is fresh. It helps to locate the fracture (Figs. 11 and 12). Variations in the ossification pattern of the xiphisternum may give the impression of fracture in the lower part of the sternum.[13] Sternal fractures are usually accompanied by trauma to the anterior part of the ribs and the costal cartilages.

The mortality rate from sternal fracture is 25%–45%. Death results not from the fracture per se but from associated intrathoracic injuries to the aorta, trachea, diaphragm, heart, or lungs.[15] Both sternal fracture and traumatic

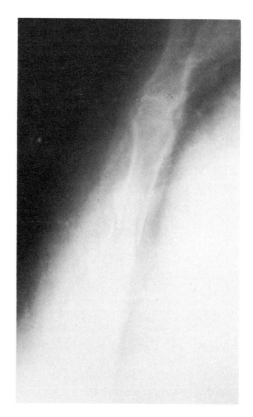

Fig. 12.   Fracture of the sternum with swelling of anterior soft tissue in a 71-year-old woman (retouched).

rupture of the aorta or a major vessel in the mediastinum produce widening of the mediastinum on the PA chest film.

The projections used in examining the sternum for fracture include the following: (1) An oblique view with the sternum near the film and its shadow superimposed on the cardiac shadow.[20] In the cooperative patient, a long exposure is preferable, because breathing blurs the underlying cardiopulmonary shadows. (2) Coned lateral view. A retrosternal hematoma is adequately seen in this position and may aid in locating the fracture. (3) AP or lateral zonography (thick-cut tomography).[18]

REFERENCES

1. Bavendam FA, Nedelman SH: Some considerations in the roentgenology of fractures and dislocations. Semin Roentgenol 1:407–436, 1966

2. Bernatz PE, Burnside AF, Clagett OT: Problems of the ruptured diaphragm. JAMA 168:877–881, 1958

3. Blatt ES, Schneider HJ, Wiot JF, Felson B: Roentgen findings in obstructed diaphragmatic hernia. Radiology 79:648, 1962

4. Burke JF: Early diagnosis of traumatic rupture of the bronchus. JAMA 181:682–686, 1962

5. Carter BN, Giuseffi J, Felson B: Traumatic diaphragmatic hernia. Am J Roentgenol 65:56, 1951

6. Chesterman JT, Satasangi PN: Rupture of the trachea and bronchi by closed injury. Thorax 21:21–27, 1966

7. Cohn R: Nonpenetrating wounds of the lungs and bronchi. Surg Clin North Am 52:585–595, 1972

8. Crawford WO Jr: Pulmonary injury in thoracic and non-thoracic trauma. Radiol Clin North Am 11:527–541, 1973

9. Eastridge CE, Hughes FA Jr, Pate JW, Cole F, Richardson R: Tracheobronchial injury caused by blunt trauma. Am Rev Respir Dis 101:230–237, 1970

10. Felson B: Chest Roentgenology. Philadelphia, WB Saunders, 1973, pp 351–359

11. Freimanis AF: Personal communication

12. Gershon-Cohen J, Hermel MB, Byrne RN, Bringhurst L: Rupture of the spleen: Roentgen diagnosis. Radiology 57:521–527, 1951

13. Golding FC: Traumatic lesions of bones and joints, in Shanks SS, Kerley P (eds): A Textbook of X-ray Diagnosis by British Authors, vol 6. Philadelphia, WB Saunders, 1971, pp 216–217

14. Grimes OF: Nonpenetrating injuries to the chest wall and esophagus. Surg Clin North Am 52:597–609, 1972

15. Harris JH Jr, Harris WH: The Radiology of Emergency Medicine. Baltimore, Williams & Wilkins, 1975, pp 218–223

16. Hill LD: Injuries of the diaphragm following blunt trauma. Surg Clin North Am 52:611–624, 1972

17. Hood RM: Traumatic diaphragmatic hernia (collective review). Ann Thorac Surg 12:311–324, 1971

18. Kattan KR: Essential knowledge about pitfalls in tomography. CRC Crit Rev Clin Radiol Nucl Med 8:329–367, 1976

19. Merrill V: Atlas of Roentgenographic Positions and Standard Radiographic Procedures. St Louis, CV Mosby, 1975, pp 164–173

20. Meschan J: An Atlas of Anatomy Basic to Radiology. Philadelphia, WB Saunders, 1975, pp 475–481

21. Orringer MB, Kirsh MV, Sloan H: Congenital and traumatic diaphragmatic hernias exclusive of the hiatus. Curr Probl Surg. Chicago, Yearbook Publishers, March 1 1975, pp 33–64

22. Peck WA Jr: Right sided diaphragmatic liver hernia following trauma. Am J Roentgenol 78:99, 1957

23. Pierce GE, Maxwell JA, Boggan MD: Special hazards of first rib fractures. J Trauma 15:264–267, 1975

24. Reynolds J, Davis JT: Injuries of the chest wall, pleura, lungs, bronchi, and esophagus. Radiol Clin North Am 4:383–401, 1966

25. Rosoff L, Cohen JL, Telfer N, Halpern M: Injuries of the spleen. Surg Clin North Am 52:667–685, 1972

26. Stevens E, Templeton AW: Traumatic nonpenetrating lung contusion. Radiology 85:247–252, 1965

27. Trackler RT, Brunkler RA: Widening of the left paravertebral pleural line on supine chest roentgenograms in free pleural effusions. Am J Roentgenol 96:1027–1034, 1966

28. Williams JR, Bonte FJ: Pulmonary damage in nonpenetrating chest injury. Radiol Clin North Am 1:439–448, 1963

29. Wiot JF: The radiologic manifestations of blunt chest trauma. JAMA 231:500–503, 1975

Shoulder

Helene Pavlov and Robert H. Freiberger

THE most common fractures of the shoulder girdle are those of the proximal humerus and humeral head, those resulting from glenohumeral dislocations, scapular and clavicular fractures, and fracture dislocations of the acromioclavicular and sternoclavicular joints. The classifications of particular injuries, their mechanisms of injury, and the optimal radiographic projections to delineate these lesions and their associated complications will be considered in this section.

FRACTURES OF THE PROXIMAL HUMERUS

Upper humeral fractures usually result from a direct blow to the shoulder or from a fall on the outstretched arm. Neer[15] provided a clinically useful classification of fractures of the proximal humerus based on the locations and the relationships of the four major fragments: the articular surface proximal to the anatomic neck, the lesser tuberosity, the greater tuberosity, and the humeral shaft. Because the fragments are held together by the rotator cuff, the joint capsule, and the intact periosteum,[16] 80% of shoulder fractures have no significant displacement. Such a nondisplaced fracture is classified as a *one-part fracture* (Fig. 1).

Displacement of one fragment constitutes a *two-part fracture,* which comprises 15% of all humeral fractures. Displacement is defined as separation of fracture fragments by at least 1 cm or 45 degrees angulation. Two-part fractures are usually unstable because of associated soft-tissue injury, most commonly involving the rotator cuff.

In a *three-part fracture,* there is displacement of two fragments. It often includes a surgical neck fracture with rotation of the head. When the greater tuberosity remains attached to the head, the supraspinatus, infraspinatus, and teres minor muscles rotate the humeral head anteriorly. If the lesser tuberosity remains attached, the humeral head is rotated posteriorly by the pull of the subscapularis muscle. The pectoralis major is responsible for anteromedial displacement of the humeral shaft.

A *four-part fracture* involves fracture of the anatomic neck of the humerus plus displacement of the lesser and the greater tuberosities.

Intraarticular fractures may produce hemarthrosis, which may then cause inferior displacement of the humeral head (Fig. 1). This displacement is called a "hanging shoulder" or a pseudosubluxation. It does not require reduction, and the deformity disappears with the resorption of the hemarthrosis. Nerve injury may cause similar displacement, but other neu-

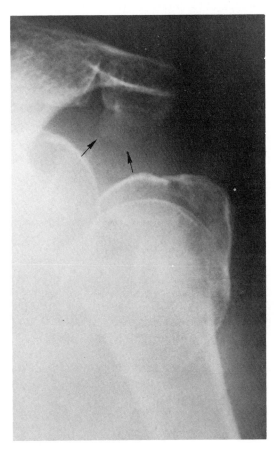

Fig. 1. Neer one-part fracture. There is comminuted fracture of the humeral head, but the fragments are not displaced. There is pseudosubluxation produced by hemarthrosis. An incidental os acromiale is present (arrows).

Helene Pavlov, M.D.: *Assistant Professor of Radiology;* Robert H. Freiberger, M.D.: *Professor of Radiology; Cornell University Medical College, The Hospital for Special Surgery, New York, N.Y.*

Reprint requests should be addressed to Dr. Helene Pavlov, Department of Radiology, The Hospital for Special Surgery, 535 East 70th Street, New York, N.Y. 10021.
© 1978 by Grune & Stratton, Inc.
0037–198X/78/1302–0003$0200/0

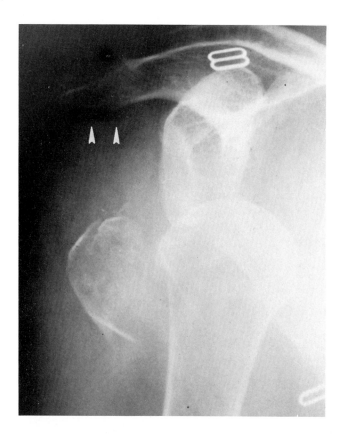

Fig. 2. Fracture dislocation of the shoulder. The fractured greater tuberosity is displaced over 1 cm, and the humerus is anteriorly dislocated. A fat-fluid level is present (arrowheads).

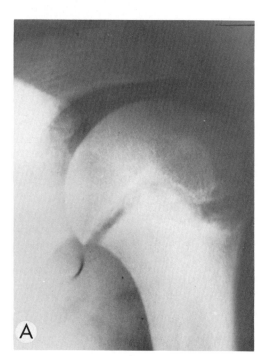

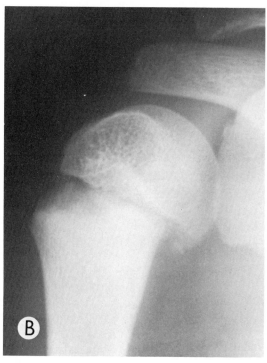

Fig. 3. Shoulder injuries in baseball pitchers. (A) The lateral aspect of the epiphyseal plate is widened, and there is irregularity of the metaphysis. This youth had pain when pitching a baseball. (B) Slipped proximal humeral epiphysis, a Salter I fracture, in a Little League pitcher.

rologic manifestations are associated. A fat–fluid level on a horizontal-beam film (Fig. 2) confirms that bone marrow fat has entered the joint and that an intraarticular fracture is present, even if it is not radiographically visible.

With fracture of the proximal humerus in a child, the fracture line usually involves the epiphysis and is described according to the Salter classification of epiphyseal injuries.[18] Epiphyseal injuries of the shoulder are associated with birth trauma, but they also occur in Little League pitchers[1,5,19] (Fig. 3) and in battered children. Proximal humeral shaft fracture in a child is usually of the pathologic variety, often through a previously asymptomatic benign bone cyst (Fig. 4).

FRACTURES RESULTING FROM DISLOCATIONS

The articular surface of the humeral head is usually fractured by shoulder dislocation. About 97% of all glenohumeral dislocations are of the anterior variety. Anterior shoulder dislocation is usually associated with the Hill-Sachs deformity.[10] This defect is a compression fracture on the posterolateral aspect of the humeral head caused by impaction against the anterior rim of the glenoid fossa. The axillary view (Fig. 5) will demonstrate the anteriorly dislocated humeral head and the mechanism of the Hill-Sachs deformity. The axillary view requires abduction and external rotation of the humerus and should never be attempted in a recently

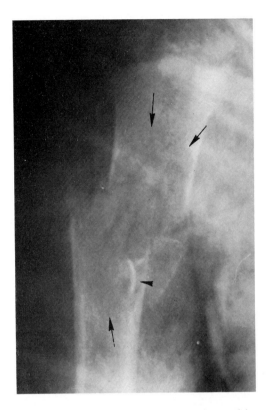

Fig. 4. Pathologic fracture through a unicameral bone cyst in the proximal humeral diaphysis (arrows) on an upright hanging cast view. A "fallen fragment" of cortical bone (arrowhead) is identified in the distal portion of the cyst. A bone fragment may fall to the most dependent part of a fluid-filled cyst, and upright or decubitus films will document its change in position.

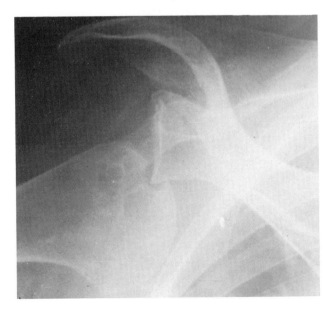

Fig. 5. Axillary view of an anteriorly dislocated shoulder demonstrates impingement of the supralateral aspect of the humeral head on the inferior glenoid rim. The Hill-Sachs defect is prominent in this patient with a history of recurrent dislocations.

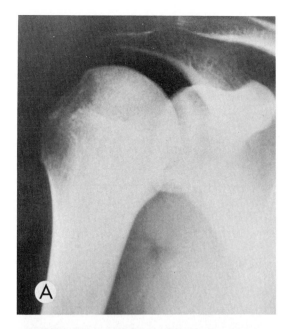

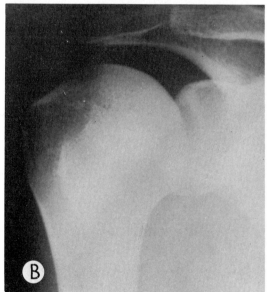

Fig. 6. (A) A Hill-Sachs defect is indicated by the flattened and irregular supralateral aspect of the humeral head on the AP view of the shoulder with the humerus internally rotated. (B) AP view in external rotation. The extent of the Hill-Sachs defect is obscured by the greater tuberosity and the intact portion of the humeral head. The acromioclavicular alignment is normal.

reduced dislocation, since this position repeats the mechanism of the initial injury and the shoulder is vulnerable to repeated dislocations.

The Hill-Sachs deformity is best detected radiographically at the superolateral aspect of the humeral head on a frontal view of the shoulder

with the humerus internally rotated (Fig. 6A). When the humerus is externally rotated, the greater tuberosity and the intact portion of the humeral head may mask the defect (Fig. 6B).

Compression fractures are found at the anteromedial aspect of the humeral head when the humerus is posteriorly dislocated. Approximately 2% of all glenohumeral dislocations are of the posterior type. This is often caused by an electric shock or an epileptic convulsion. Posterior dislocation is frequently missed at physical examination because it produces no clearly visible or palpable deformity. About half of them are missed at the first roentgen examination as well. The difficulty in roentgen diagnosis of a posterior dislocation arises in part because the humeral head is not completely displaced posteriorly and medially to the glenoid fossa, and also because the glenoid is so shaped that the routine AP view of the shoulder does not demonstrate it tangentially. The humeral head normally overlaps the posterior three-fourths of the glenoid fossa on the AP film. With posterior dislocation, the humeral head is displaced laterally, so that overlap with the glenoid fossa is reduced, but this reduction is subtle and easily missed (Fig. 7A). Lewis[14] suggested a 30-degree posterior oblique view of the involved shoulder to produce a tangential view of the articular surface of the glenoid fossa and permit direct analysis of the glenohumeral alignment. On this view, the posteriorly dislocated humeral head obliterates the normally unobstructed joint space (Fig. 7B).

The tuberosities are vulnerable to fracture during dislocation. Anterior dislocations are commonly associated with fracture of the greater tuberosity (Fig. 2), and posterior dislocations are commonly associated with fracture of the lesser tuberosity. Fracture of the greater tuberosity also occurs with the rare inferior dislocation of the glenohumeral joint, in which the superior articular surface of the humeral head is displaced directly inferior to the glenoid rim. When this dislocation is associated with fixed elevation of the arm, it is called *luxatio erecta*[17] (Fig. 8). It usually results from a fall on the abducted arm. In such a fall, the arm acts as a lever, and the acromion acts as a fulcrum to push the humeral head out of the joint and under the glenoid. The luxatio erecta may be accompanied by fracture of the acromion process

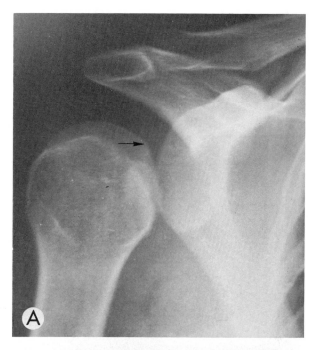

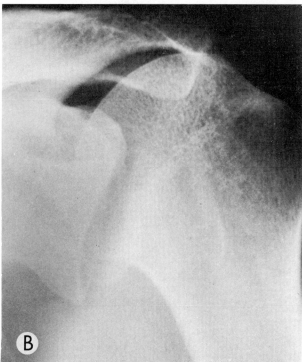

Fig. 7. Posterior dislocation of the shoulder. (A) Routine AP view of the shoulder. The humeral head is laterally displaced and barely overlaps the glenoid fossa. The smooth articular surface of the humeral head is interrupted (arrow), and the medial surface is flattened and irregular because of a compression fracture. (B) Posterior shoulder dislocation confirmed by a tangential view of the glenoid (30–40 degree posterior oblique of the affected shoulder). The glenohumeral joint space is absent, and the humeral head overlaps the glenoid posterosuperiorly.

or the inferior glenoid fossa, rotator cuff tear, and neurovascular damage.

The scapula may be fractured in any dislocation. The inferior lip of the glenoid fossa is occasionally fractured by anterior dislocation, and this is called a Bankart lesion[3] (Fig. 9). When the fracture involves only the articular cartilage, it will not be evident on plain films. In such instances a double contrast shoulder arthrogram will delineate the abnormality.[7,9]

Two films at right angles are generally deemed necessary for evaluating all fractures,

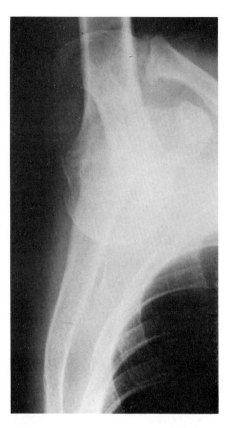

Fig. 8. Luxatio erecta. The arm is elevated, and the humeral head is inferiorly dislocated. The greater tuberosity is fractured.

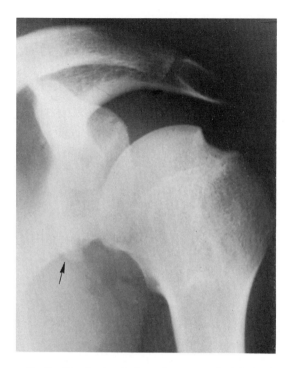

Fig. 9. The Bankart lesion, a fracture at the inferior rim of the glenoid, is identified by the presence of an osseous fragment (arrow). A Hill-Sachs defect is also evident. This patient had a history of multiple anterior shoulder dislocations, one of which had recently been reduced.

and the shoulder joint should be no exception. The transscapular view and either a frontal or tangential view should be obtained. The transscapular view is valuable for diagnosis of a posterior dislocation and to detail scapular anatomy. This view is obtained by placing the patient in a 30–45-degree anterior oblique position, turned toward the affected side, with the central ray parallel and directed through the scapular blade.[17] The intersection of the acromion, coracoid, and body of the scapula form a Y in this projection (Fig. 10). The humeral head, if normally located, is superimposed over the Y. The integrity of the coracoid process and acromion process and acromioclavicular alignment can be readily evaluated in this view.

Complications Associated With Glenohumeral Injuries

Shoulder fractures and fracture dislocations may cause a variety of complications. Avascular necrosis of the head of the humerus may follow any fracture involving the anatomic neck. Adhe-

sive capsulitis or "frozen shoulder" may be a sequel to trauma and immobilization. A localized area of radiolucency of the humeral head on plain radiographs may arouse suspicion of adhesive capsulitis, but an arthrogram demonstrating a tight capsule provides a more accurate diagnosis.[13]

Nonunion of the greater tuberosity and myositis ossificans about the shoulder are rare complications of shoulder fracture. Nonunion of the greater tuberosity may produce limitation of external rotation and abduction of the arm. Myositis ossificans usually does not limit range of motion. It eventually disappears.

Chronic rotator cuff tear is caused by a degenerative process and can be detected on plain films because the humeral head migrates superiorly and abuts on the undersurface of the acromion. The undersurface of the acromion will be faceted and concave (Fig. 11).

Acute rotator cuff tear may occur as an isolated injury or with shoulder dislocation. Acute rotator cuff tear shows no abnormality on routine films; thus the roentgen diagnosis is best made by arthrography[13] (Fig. 12).

Although accurate diagnosis of a rotator cuff

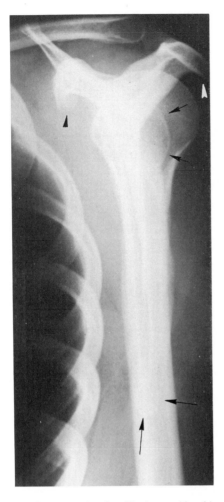

Fig. 10. Transscapular view. The humeral head is super-imposed on the glenoid fossa (short arrows). The coracoid process (black arrowhead), acromion process (white arrowhead), and the scapular blade (long arrows) form a Y. This view can also be used for evaluation of the acromioclavicular joint.

tear can be made by single contrast arthrogram, the size of the tear, the edge of the torn cuff, and the intraarticular portion of the biceps tendon may also be demonstrated by double contrast shoulder arthrography.[8,9]

FRACTURES OF THE SCAPULA

Injuries to the scapula are the result of direct trauma. Fractures of the body and the spine of the scapula usually are undisplaced because they are protected by bulky muscle attachments. Fractures are best examined on transscapular and frontal views (Fig. 13). Complications are rare, but injury to the axillary artery and brachial plexus has been reported.

Fracture of the scapular neck occurs as a

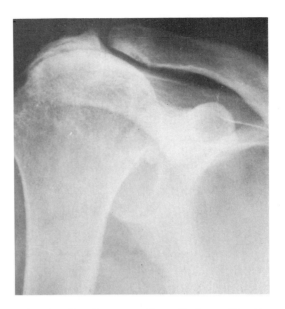

Fig. 11. Chronic rotator cuff tear. The humeral head has migrated superiorly. The acromion process is narrowed, and its undersurface has remodeled to form a concave "articulation" with the humeral head.

consequence of a direct blow to the shoulder, in association with surgical neck fracture of the humerus. The glenoid rim of the scapula is fractured in 20% of patients with fracture dislocation of the shoulder, as has been previously discussed. Occasionally, violent throwing action with strong triceps contraction will also produce avulsion of the inferior lip of the glenoid.[4]

The acromion process is fractured by a direct downward blow to the shoulder. It is important not to confuse this with an os acromiale (Fig. 1), which is a normal variant and is bilateral in 60% of patients. Occasionally the ossification centers of the coracoid process are misinterpreted as a fracture in the adolescent[12] (Fig. 14).

FRACTURES OF THE CLAVICLE

The clavicle is the only osseous connection between the upper extremity and the trunk, so that clavicle fracture results in drooping of the shoulder anteriorly because of muscle pull and inferiorly because of the weight of the arm. Fracture of the clavicle is a frequent birth and childhood injury. Any direct blow or fall on the lateral aspect of the clavicle can cause it. Clavicle fractures involve the middle third in 80%, the lateral third in 15%, and the medial third in 5% of cases.

Fractures of the lateral portion of the clavicle are divided into three types: (1) undisplaced

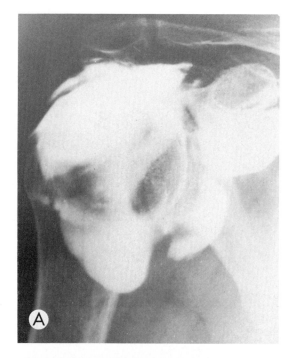

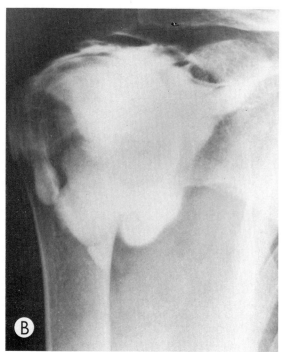

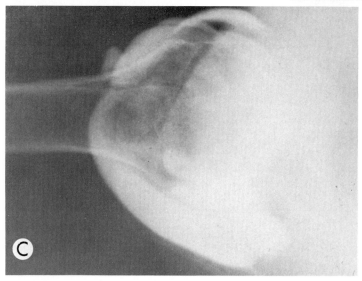

Fig. 12. Abnormal single contrast shoulder arthrogram, documenting a torn rotator cuff. The humerus is in (A) internal and (B) external rotation. The contrast is seen in the location of the rotator cuff, above the humeral head and below the acromion process in both views, and it extends over the greater tuberosity on the external rotation view. (C) The axillary view demonstrates contrast medium crossing the humeral shaft.

fracture, (2) displaced fracture with the medial portion displaced posteriorly by the pull of the trapezius muscle and the lateral fragment displaced anteriorly and inferiorly, and (3) articular surface fracture, which occurs at the acromioclavicular joint and occasionally at the sternoclavicular joint. The articular fractures are often overlooked and result in pain and arthritic changes.

Fracture of the medial aspect of the clavicle usually results from direct trauma.

Complications of Clavicle Fractures

In children, clavicular fractures heal rapidly and without sequelae. In adults, these fractures are usually the result of more violent trauma, and although most heal without difficulty, there may be complications. Callus formation during healing may be so exuberant that it causes neurovascular compromise by compression of nerves and vessels against the first rib. The excessive callus may also be cosmetically objectionable. Malunion or nonunion, although rare,

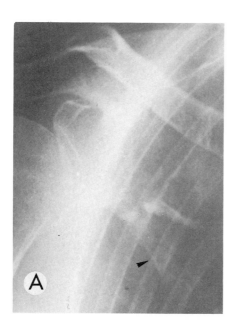
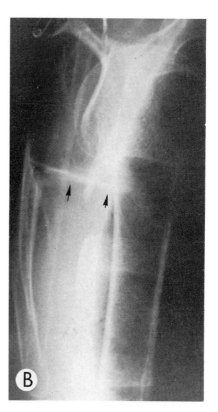

Fig. 13.   Fracture of body of scapula. (A) Frontal view of the shoulder demonstrates two linear densities in the scapular body. Note lateral scapular margin (arrowhead). (B) Transscapular view delineates the fracture (arrows). The fracture fragments are displaced at right angles to the body of the scapula and correspond to the densities present on the frontal view.

may produce severe disfigurement and may be responsible for a painful shoulder. Severe trauma may also cause laceration of the subclavian vessels or brachial plexus by displaced fragments, requiring emergency surgical treatment.

Arthritis is the most common sequela, and it follows unsuspected ligamentous tears at the acromioclavicular or the sternoclavicular joints.

ACROMIOCLAVICULAR INJURIES

Acromioclavicular dislocation results from falling onto the shoulder with arm adducted or falling onto the outstretched arm. The force is transmitted through the humeral head to the acromion process.

The region of the acromioclavicular joint is usually overpenetrated on routine films of the shoulder; thus specific views of this area should be requested. A 15-degree cranial tilt of the central ray will project the area clearly. In the normal shoulder, the inferior surfaces of the acromion process and of the distal clavicle are in alignment (Figs. 6, 9, and 10). The average

normal distance between the superior surface of the coracoid process and the inferior aspect of the clavicle is 1.1–1.3 cm; a difference of 3–4 mm or more indicates coracoclavicular liga-

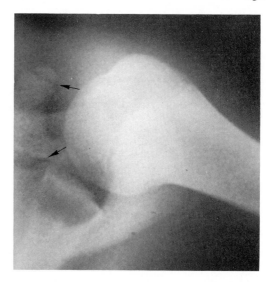

Fig. 14.   Ossification centers of the coracoid process (arrows).

ment disruption. Angulation of the tube will project the coracoid and clavicle differently; thus comparison of the injured shoulder with the normal shoulder is essential for accurately determining these measurements and the alignment. Acromioclavicular fracture-dislocation can be detected by a weight-holding film. This tests the integrity of the coracoclavicular ligament. Views should include both shoulders, with and without 5–15-lb weights suspended from the patient's wrists or hands.[17]

Acromioclavicular joint injuries are classified by the degree of involvement of the acromioclavicular and coracoclavicular ligaments.[2] Type I acromioclavicular joint injury clinically corresponds to a mild sprain in which the acromioclavicular ligament is stretched but not disrupted and the coracoclavicular ligament is intact. Acromioclavicular alignment is normal with and without weight-holding. The joint is clinically stable. There is no evidence of joint space widening or irregularity on the initial films.

Type II acromioclavicular joint injury corresponds clinically to a moderate sprain in which the acromioclavicular ligament is torn and the coracoclavicular ligaments are stretched. Radiographs reveal widening of the acromioclavicular joint with slight elevation of the lateral aspect of the clavicle. The clavicle elevation may increase with stress films, but it will be less than half the width of the clavicle. This represents an acromioclavicular subluxation.

Type III injury corresponds clinically to a severe sprain with rupture of both the coracoclavicular and acromioclavicular ligaments. Occasionally the coracoclavicular ligaments remain intact, but the coracoid process is avulsed. The lateral aspect of the clavicle is elevated above and may override the acromion process. The joint space is widened. This represents an acromioclavicular dislocation.

STERNOCLAVICULAR JOINT INJURIES

Sternoclavicular dislocation is rare and usually is caused by an automobile or football accident. The sternoclavicular joint is injured by a direct blow to it or by impact at the shoulder with the force transmitted along the long axis of the clavicle. The sternoclavicular joint is difficult to examine roentgenographically; thus the initial diagnosis and subsequent treatment are usually determined by clinical palpation. Adequate radiographic examination may require angulation of the tube 40 degrees cephalad for an apical lordotic view of the sterno-clavicular joints,[11] a stereoscopic technique, or tomography. To permit comparison, both sternoclavicular joints must be included in the examination.

Dislocation of the clavicle anterior to the manubrium is the most common type. Posterior displacement is very rare (Fig. 15), but it is potentially dangerous because there are vital structures behind the sternoclavicular joint, including the pulmonary arteries, subclavian vessels, jugular vein, phrenic nerve, and trachea, that might be injured.

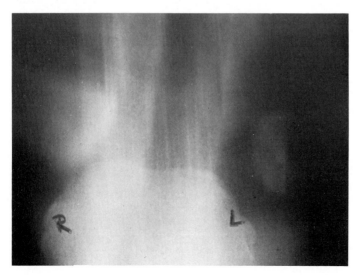

Fig. 15. Tomogram of the sternoclavicular joints reveals posterior dislocation on the right.

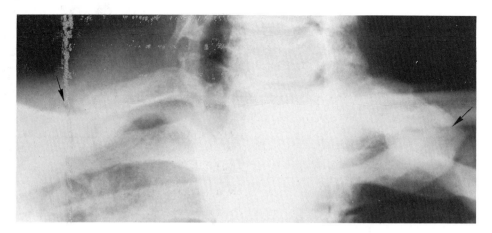

Fig. 16.   Bilateral fractures of the first ribs (arrows).

RIB FRACTURES

A fracture-like defect in the posterior portion of an otherwise normally formed first rib may represent an acute or stress fracture. These occur when an occupation requires lifting heavy weights or involves excessive overhead use of the arms. They may be bilateral. Most of these fractures are asymptomatic, although a sticking pain has been described. The bone adjacent to the fracture line may become sclerotic, and callus may be present. Follow-up examination usually shows complete healing[6] (Fig. 16).

Pseudofractures, called Looser zones, are narrow bands of radiolucency oriented perpendicularly or obliquely to the bone surface. They are usually symmetric bilaterally and are pathognomonic of osteomalacia. The upper ribs, lateral scapula, and proximal humeri are common sites of pseudofracture.

RADIOGRAPHIC TECHNIQUES FOR
SHOULDER EXAMINATIONS

The radiographic examination of the shoulder should be modified according to the nature of the suspected injury and the patient's physical condition. An adequate radiographic examination of the shoulder is best performed with the patient standing or sitting and the arm dependent, and includes AP views with the humerus in internal and external rotation. Evaluation of osseous integrity, of the Hill-Sachs and Bankart defects, of glenohumeral and acromioclavicular alignment, and of soft tissues for hemarthrosis, fat–fluid level, and calcification is possible from these two AP

views. If necessary, the two views can be taken with the patient supine.

Following shoulder trauma, a patient may be reluctant or unable to move the arm, or it may have been immobilized by a sling and swathe dressing by the referring clinician. By modifying the technique, the internal and external rotation views can still be obtained with the patient supine or standing. In the routine AP view of the shoulder, the humerus will be in internal rotation. Without moving the injured arm, the external rotation view can be obtained by rotating the patient 30 to 45 degrees posteriorly toward the affected shoulder.

When a fracture of the humeral shaft below the neck is suspected, a pair of right angle films should be taken. An AP view of the humerus in either internal or external rotation and a transthoracic lateral view will adequately detail displacement and angulation of the fracture fragments. The transthoracic lateral view is not helpful when the suspected injury involves the humeral head or a glenohumeral dislocation because the ribs obscure detail. In these cases, a transscapular view is preferred.

An anterior dislocation may be detected on the usual AP view by medial inferior displacement of the humeral head. The presence of a fat–fluid level on a horizontal beam film indicates an intraarticular fracture, probably of the greater tuberosity, which may not be initially evident on the radiograph.

A posterior dislocation, as previously discussed, may have subtle roentgen findings, but it can be diagnosed if suspected. Either a tangential view of the glenohumeral joint or a transscapular view of the scapula will confirm or exclude the diagnosis. The positioning for these views has been discussed above.

An axillary view may be helpful to evaluate the shoulder, but a patient with a dislocated shoulder may not be able to cooperate; if the shoulder had been recently reduced, the arm should not be abducted without the referring clinician present, as recurrence of the dislocation may occur.

In evaluating the scapula for a fracture, two right angle films are necessary: a transscapular view and a frontal view. The frontal view of the scapula is obtained with the patient in a posterior oblique position, turned 45 degrees toward the affected side, with the cones opened to include the entire scapula. The coracoid and acromion processes are also visible on these views. If an additional view is desired, an oblique view of the scapula with the humerus abducted may be obtained as an additional view of the shoulder.

The clavicle can usually be evaluated on simple routine PA or AP views, erect or horizontal. The acromioclavicular area is occasionally overpenetrated on routine shoulder films, and if this is the area of concern, the factors should be adjusted appropriately. The tube should be angled cephalad approximately 15 degrees, and comparison views with the opposite side should be obtained. Weight-holding films may depict a type II acromioclavicular injury not evident without the added stress.

The sternoclavicular joints should also be evaluated with comparison views of the opposite side. Demonstration of a dislocation of the sternoclavicular joint usually requires tomography. A tomogram can also help determine if both clavicles are in focus at the same level. Stereoscopic, oblique, apical lordotic, and lateral views of the manubrium may be helpful in visualizing the sternoclavicular joint.

ACKNOWLEDGMENTS

Our grateful appreciation goes to Nidia M. Rodriguez for her patience and skill in typing the multiple versions of this manuscript and to Jill Spiller for her constructive editorial review.

REFERENCES

1. Adams JE: Little league shoulder: osteochondrosis of the proximal humeral epiphysis in boy baseball pitchers. Calif Med 105:22–25, 1966

2. Allman FL Jr: Fractures and ligamentous injuries of the clavicle and its articulation. J Bone Joint Surg [Am] 49:774–784, 1967

3. Bankart ASB: Recurrent or habitual dislocation of the shoulder-joint. Br Med J 2:1132–1133, 1923

4. Bowerman JW, McDonnell EJ: Radiology of athletic injuries: baseball. Radiology 116:611–615, 1975

5. Dotter WE: Little leaguer's shoulder—A fracture of the proximal epiphyseal cartilage of the humerus due to baseball pitching. Guthrie Clinic Bull 23:68, 1953

6. Freiberger RH, Mayer V: Ununited bilateral fatigue fractures of the first ribs. A case report and review of the literature. J Bone Joint Surg [Am] 46:615–618, 1964

7. Ghelman B: Double contrast arthrography of the shoulder in the evaluation of the cartilaginous labrum of the glenoid. (submitted for publication).

8. Ghelman B, Goldman AB: The double contrast shoulder arthrogram: evaluation of rotatory cuff tears. Radiology 124:251–254, 1977

9. Goldman AB, Ghelman B: The double contrast shoulder arthrogram. A review of 158 studies. Radiology (in press)

10. Hill HA, Sachs MD: The grooved defect of the humeral head. A frequently unrecognized complication of dislocations of the shoulder joint. Radiology 35:690–700, 1940

11. Hobbs DW: Sternoclavicular joint: a new axial radiographic view. Radiology 90:801, 1968

12. Keats RE: An Atlas of Normal Roentgen Variants that May Simulate Disease. Chicago, Year Book, 1975, p 119

13. Killoran PJ, Marcove RC, Freiberger RH: Shoulder Arthrography. Am J Roentgenol 103: 658–668, 1968

14. Lewis RW: The Joints of the Extremities: A Radiographic Study. Springfield Ill, Charles C Thomas, 1955

15. Neer CS II: Displaced proximal humeral fractures. Part I. Classification and evaluation. J Bone Joint Surg [Am] 52:1077–1089, 1970

16. Neer CS II: Part I: Fractures about the shoulder, in Rockwood CA, Jr., Green DP (eds): Fractures, vol 1. Philadelphia, JB Lippincott, 1975 p 585

17. Rockwood CA: Part II: Dislocations about the shoulder, in Rockwood CA Jr, Green DP (eds): Fractures, vol 1, Philadelphia, JB Lippincott, 1975, p 624

18. Salter RB, Harris WR: Injuries involving the epiphyseal plate. J Bone Joint Surg [Am] 45:587–622, 1963

19. Torg JS, Pollack H, Sweterlitsch P: The effect of competitive pitching on the shoulders and elbows of preadolescent baseball players. Pediatrics 49:267–272, 1972

Elbow

Lee F. Rogers

INTERPRETATION of radiographs obtained for evaluation of elbow trauma is at times difficult. The difficulty arises from the combination of the complex anatomy and the obscure nature of some injuries. The presence of multiple epiphyseal and apophyseal growth centers and their variability makes evaluation of elbow injuries in children a particular challenge. Errors can be avoided by an orderly approach to the roentgenographic analysis, utilizing well-defined anatomic relationships, tables of the growth center ossification sequence, and knowledge of the statistical frequency of injury at various sites. It is quite important to know the circumstances or mechanism of injury and the pertinent physical findings. Unfortunately these are frequently not available or incomplete. It is an excellent practice to examine the patient personally. Knowing where the patient hurts and the nature and degree of limitation of motion is most helpful. "Fell from ladder at home this afternoon" is not a particularly helpful history. It would be much better to read, "Injured elbow in fall from a height; pain laterally; limitation of pronation and supination." Undoubtedly the obscure fracture of the radial head would be more readily and confidently identified. The absence of such a succinct statement is as much a reflection of the referring clinician's lack of knowledge regarding the patient's condition as it is a disregard for the requirements of good roentgenographic interpretation.

ANATOMY

The humeral shaft flares to form the medial and lateral condyles. The medial is the more prominent of the two. The flexor pronator muscles of the forearm arise from the medial epicondyle, and the extensor muscles of the forearm arise from the lateral epicondyle. The distal articular surface of the humerus is a continuation of the condyles and forms two distinct articulations. The grooved medial surface is termed the trochlea, and it articulates with the ulna. The rounded lateral surface, the capitellum, articulates with the radial head. The boundary between the two is the lateral trochlear ridge. Above the trochlea there are opposing depressions in the anterior and posterior surfaces, termed the coronoid and olecranon fossa, respectively.

The concave articulating surface of the ulna is the trochlear notch. The anterior margin of the notch is a triangular projection, the coronoid process, which serves as the insertion of the brachialis muscle. The posterior margin of the notch is formed by the olecranon, which serves as the insertion of the triceps muscle.

The radial head contains a shallow depression that articulates with the capitellum. Just distal to it, the radius constricts to form the neck and then expands to form the radial tuberosity, which serves as the attachment for the biceps tendon. The annular ligament encircles the radial head and secures the radius to the ulna.

ROENTGENOGRAPHIC VIEWS

The initial examination consists of AP and lateral projections of the injured side (Fig. 1A and B). The AP view should be obtained with the forearm supinated and the elbow in as full extension as possible. The lateral view should be obtained in 90-degree flexion of the elbow. Internal and external oblique projections with the forearm in full extension are helpful in disclosing otherwise inapparent injuries. They are of particular value in the identification of subtle fractures of the radial head (Fig. 1C) and the coronoid process of the ulna (Fig. 2). Comparison views of the opposite side should be obtained if there is any question concerning the presence or position of apophyseal and epiphyseal growth centers or the normal appearance of some bony structure.

Lee F. Rogers, M.D.: *Professor and Chairman, Department of Radiology, Northwestern University Medical School, Chicago, Ill.*

Reprint requests should be addressed to Dr. Lee F. Rogers, Department of Radiology, Northwestern University Medical School, 303 East Chicago Avenue, Chicago, Ill. 60611.

© 1978 by Grune & Stratton, Inc.

0037–198X/78/1302–0004$0200/0

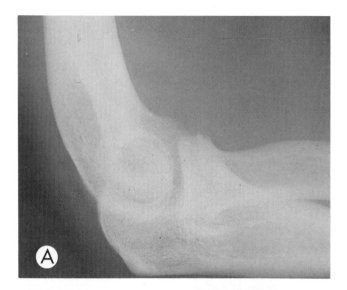

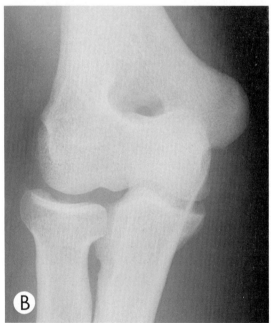

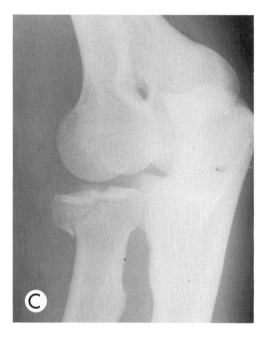

Fig. 1.   Fracture of head of radius in an adult: (A) Lateral view. There is no evidence of fracture. No fat pad is seen. (B) AP view. Depression of a segment of the radial head is suggested. (C) External oblique view. The fracture is obvious.

ROENTGENOGRAPHIC FINDINGS

It is important to analyze, not just simply to view the radiographs. To analyze implies a search for specific findings or clues, asking specific questions, and looking at specific sites that have the greatest likelihood of showing significant findings.

Granted, in many cases the injury is immediately obvious, as with a comminuted frac-

ture of the humeral condyles, and analysis may prove unnecessary. However, if the analysis stops with the recognition of an obvious fracture of the proximal ulna, there is a real chance that an associated dislocation of the proximal radius may be overlooked (Fig. 3). A disciplined approach significantly decreases the chance of oversight of subtle injuries and thereby increases confidence in the interpretation.

Analysis of roentgenograms of the injured

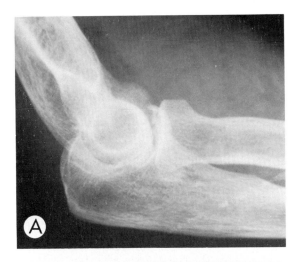

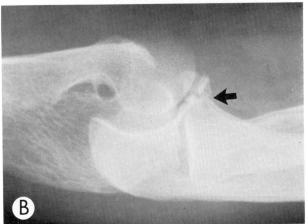

Fig. 2.   Fracture of coronoid process of ulna in an adult: (A) Lateral view. The fracture is not well seen. (B) Internal oblique view. The fracture is well demonstrated (arrow).

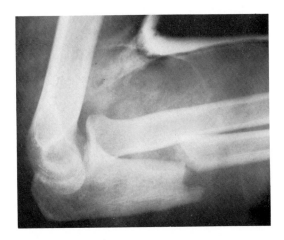

Fig. 3.   Monteggia fracture in an adult. Fracture of the proximal third of the ulna was recognized, and the arm was placed in a cast. Note the persistent anterior dislocation of the radial head, which was overlooked.

elbow should include the following: a search for fat pads; study of the anterior humeral and radiocapitellar lines to determine specific anatomic relationships; identification of the presence and proper position of ossification centers; a specific search for fractures of known high frequency.

The fat pad sign was first described by Norell[14] in 1954. A thin layer of fat overlies both the anterior and posterior aspects of the elbow joint capsule. The posterior fat pad lies in the shallow intercondylar depression on the posterior surface of the humerus and therefore is invisible on the normal lateral radiograph. On the other hand, the anterior fat pad is seen normally. It lies anterior to the coronoid fossa, extending inferiorly in an oblique line from the anterior humeral cortex.

In the presence of joint effusion, the posterior fat pad is visible on the lateral roentgenogram of the elbow, since it is displaced posteriorly

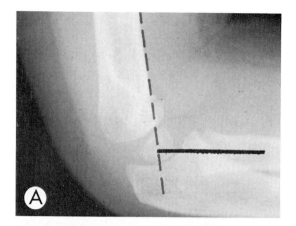

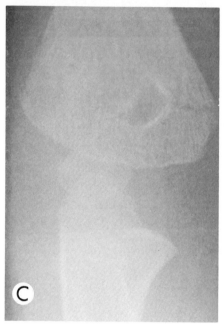

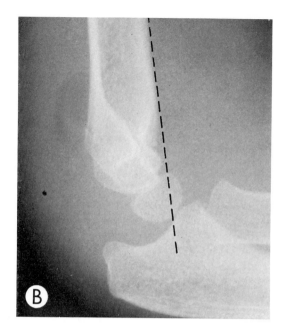

Fig. 4. Supracondylar fracture in a 5-year-old child: (A) Lateral view of normal side. The anterior humeral line (broken line) passes through the middle third of the capitellum. The radiocapitellar line (solid line) passes through the center of the capitellum. (B) Lateral view of injured side. A posterior fat pad sign is present. The anterior humeral line passes through the anterior third of the capitellum. A faint fracture line is present in the condylar region. (C) Injured side, AP view. An undisplaced fracture is present. Only the medial condylar component of the fracture line is well visualized.

(Fig. 4B). The anterior fat pad becomes more nearly perpendicular to the anterior humeral cortex. A visible posterior fat pad is a more reliable index of joint effusion than a perpendicularly oriented anterior fat pad. Elbow joint distension of any origin (hemorrhagic, inflammatory, or traumatic) will give rise to a positive fat pad sign, so the fat pad sign is not specific for trauma. The traumatic variety is due to a fracture that extends into the joint surface, allowing both blood and marrow content to collect within and to expand the joint. Over 90% of children and adolescents with a posterior fat pad sign prove to have a demonstrable fracture either initially or on follow-up examination.[1,2,12] The sign is usually present in children and adolescents. The sign is less frequently seen in the adult, and therefore its absence cannot be used to exclude a fracture. If a posterior fat pad sign is demonstrated in the injured adult elbow, however, the likelihood of fracture is high.

The articular surfaces of the distal humerus are not in direct alignment with the humeral shaft. They are offset anteriorly, forming an angle of approximately 140 degrees with the midshaft on the lateral roentgenogram. This angle is not easily measured. A line drawn on the lateral radiograph along the anterior surface of the humeral cortex and extended through the elbow joint, the anterior humeral line, serves as a satisfactory index of this angulation.[12] Normally the extension of this line passes through the middle third of the capitellum. In the presence of a supracondylar fracture, the anterior humeral line passes through the anterior third of the capitellum or entirely anterior to it. This is useful in the evaluation of supracondylar fractures in young children (Fig. 4). These are frequently greenstick fractures wherein the fracture line is not obvious.

A line bisecting the proximal radial shaft should always pass through the capitellum on every radiographic view.[17,19,20] This is termed the radiocapitellar line and confirms articulation between the radial head and the capitellum (Fig. 4A). If the line fails to pass through the capitellum, dislocation of the radial head is indicated. This is of particular value in recognizing the dislocation component of a Monteggia fracture (Fig. 3).

At birth the entire distal humerus is comprised of cartilage and contains no centers of ossification. The distal articular surfaces of the humerus consist predominantly of cartilage until the age of 11 or 12 years, so that the configuration and position of the articular surfaces must be surmised from the visible ossification centers. There are four ossification centers in the distal humerus[5,13,15] (Fig. 5). The first to appear is the capitellum at age 3 to 6 months. The medial epicondyle appears at age 5 to 7 years, and the trochlea at age 9 to 10 years. The last to appear is the lateral epicondyle at age 9 to 13 years. The centers appear earlier in females than in males. They fuse between the ages of 14 and 16 years, except for the medial epicondyle, which may not fuse until age 18 or 19. The ossification center for the radial head appears at age 3 to 6 years, and the olecranon center of the ulna at 6 to 10 years. The centers are generally smooth in outline and arise from a single focus,

with the exception of the trochlea, which is frequently irregular in outline and often arises from more than one center.

STATISTICAL FREQUENCY OF INJURY

As already stated, awareness of the most common sites of injury aids considerably in the search for potential fractures, since the position and course of fracture lines tend to be repetitive.

Supracondylar fracture accounts for approximately 60% of all elbow fractures in children and is by far the most common.[15,19,21] Fracture of the lateral condyle accounts for 15%, and separation of the medial epicondylar ossification center accounts for 10%. Fracture of the olecranon, separation of the proximal radial epiphysis, dislocation of the elbow, and Monteggia fracture account for most of the remainder.

Fracture of the radial head or neck is the most common injury in adults.[6] Dislocation, Monteggia fracture, and fracture of the olecranon are also relatively common. In contradistinction to the situation with children, fracture of the distal humerus is relatively uncommon.

SPECIFIC INJURIES

Distal Humerus

Fracture of the distal humerus in adults rarely poses a diagnostic problem. The fracture may be supracondylar or may involve either or both condyles. Comminuted fractures are either Y- or T-shaped, a vertical fracture line extending from the region of the trochlea and then branching to involve both condyles.

On rare occasions, a portion of the capitellum is avulsed. The resultant fragment is usually not evident on the frontal projection but is found on the lateral roentgenogram lying just above the radial head and coronoid process of the ulna (Fig. 6). Osteochondral fracture[6] of the joint surface occasionally occurs from the capitellum and is manifest by a sliver of bone of variable size within the joint space. The site of origin can seldom be identified radiologically.

Avulsion fracture of the supracondylar process[5] may occur (Fig. 7), and it should not be misinterpreted as a separate center of ossification for this atavistic bony process.

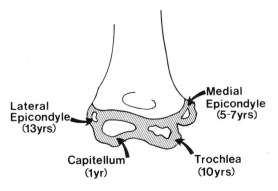

Lateral Epicondyle (13yrs)

Medial Epicondyle (5-7yrs)

Capitellum (1yr)

Trochlea (10yrs)

Fig. 5. Normal ossification sequence of growth centers of distal humerus.

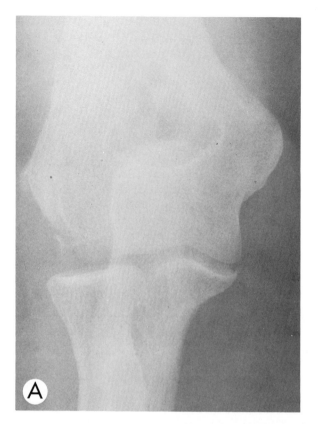

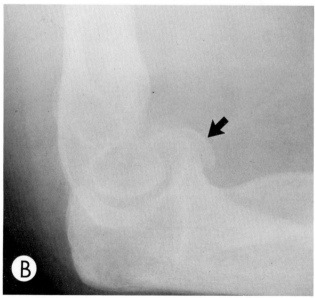

Fig. 6. Fracture of capitellum of humerus in an adult. (A) AP view. Slight irregularity of the capitellum is identified. (B) Lateral view. The capitellar fragment (arrow) is displaced proximally, typical of this type of fracture.

The most common fracture of the elbow in children is the *supracondylar fracture*.[6,15] The fracture line actually extends transversely across the condyles and through the coronoid and olecranon fossae and should thus probably be designated as a transcondylar fracture, but common usage dictates otherwise (Fig. 4). It is the result of a hyperextension injury incurred by falling on the outstretched hand. The distal fragment is displaced posteriorly. Most are complete fractures, and the diagnosis is usually obvious; however, approximately 25% are of a

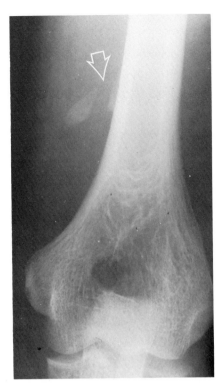

Fig. 7. Fracture of supracondylar process of the humerus (arrow), the result of a direct blow.

greenstick variety, and the radiographic findings may be subtle. A posterior fat pad sign is almost always present. The fracture either eliminates or reduces the normal volar angulation of the distal articular surface. This loss of angulation is detected by demonstrating that the anterior humeral line passes anterior to or through the anterior third of the capitellum. The fracture line is often difficult to identify on the AP projection. On the lateral projection, disruption of the anterior humeral cortex is often present.

Fracture of the lateral condyle is a Salter-Harris type IV epiphyseal injury.[9,16,22] The fracture splits the epiphysis and separates off a portion of the adjacent metaphysis (Fig. 8). It accounts for 15% of all elbow injuries in children. The fracture extends diagonally from the trochlea notch to the lateral metaphysis. This separates off a fragment containing the capitellum and a flake of metaphyseal bone. The extensors of the forearm are attached to this fragment, and therefore it is commonly displaced posteriorly and inferiorly by muscle traction. The radiocapitellar line is thus disrupted in

one or more planes. These fractures almost universally require open reduction and pin fixation to prevent subsequent angular deformity.[7]

Separation of the medial epicondylar ossification center is the result of a stress placed on the flexor pronator tendon attached to the ossification center. The avulsed fragment is displaced distally. The stress may be created by a valgus force on the elbow or by tension within the flexor pronator muscles. The latter mechanism accounts for avulsion of the medial epicondylar ossification center described in young baseball pitchers, termed Little Leaguer elbow.[4] The injury is usually obvious on the AP projection. When there is minimal displacement, a comparison view of the opposite side may be necessary for confirmation.

On occasion, the avulsed fragment is sufficiently displaced to become entrapped in the medial portion of the joint.[5,10,15] This may not be readily apparent unless one looks for it (Fig. 9). To avoid this error, always identify the presence and position of the medial epicondylar ossification center when analyzing prereduction and postreduction films of the injured elbow in children and adolescents. The entrapped fragment may be mistaken for the trochlear ossification center prior to its initial appearance at age 10. These avulsions are commonly associated with elbow dislocation in children. The center frequently becomes entrapped as a result of reduction of the dislocation.

Radius

As stated, fracture involving the head and neck of the radius is the most common elbow fracture in adults.[6] It occurs as a result of a fall on the outstretched hand, which creates an impaction of the radial head against the capitellum. The elbow is frequently forced into valgus, and the lateral margin of the radial head is therefore most likely fractured. When the fragments are displaced, the diagnosis is obvious. Frequently the fractured fragment is not displaced, and the fracture line may then be obscure and not readily visualized on the AP or lateral projections. The clinical clue to the presence of the fracture is inability to pronate or supinate the forearm. Oblique views are frequently necessary to disclose these inapparent fractures (Fig. 1). The fracture line is commonly located on the lateral aspect of the

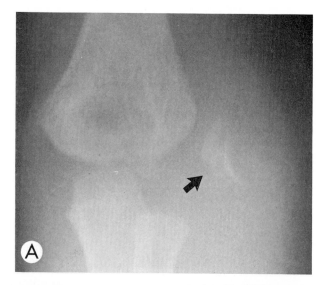

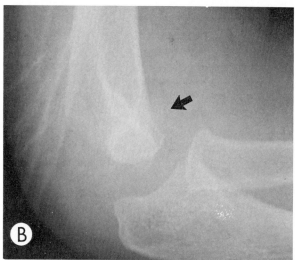

Fig. 8. Fracture of the lateral condyle, Salter type IV, in a 4-year-old child: (A) AP view. A portion of the capitellum (arrow) and an attached metaphyseal fragment are displaced laterally and rotated. (B) Lateral view. The displaced fragment (arrow) is difficult to see.

joint surface and is vertically oriented. The cortex of the peripheral margin of the radial head is disrupted, and the fragment is frequently slightly depressed.

Impaction fracture of the radial neck is best visualized on the lateral projection. Normally the anterior cortex of the radial head forms a gentle concave curve as it rises to the base of the radial head. Impaction fracture eliminates this curve and creates an abrupt step-off between the radial head and neck. On the frontal projection, this fracture may be visualized as a line of increased density at the base of the radial head.

In children and adolescents, fracture involving the joint surface of the radial head is uncommon, but separation of the proximal radial epiphysis is relatively frequent.[11,16] Most are

Salter-Harris type II injuries, wherein the fracture line lies in the growth plate and then turns to separate off a corner of the metaphysis. This metaphyseal fragment is usually situated laterally. At times there is no displacement of the radial epiphysis, and it is necessary to identify a fracture line within the radial metaphysis to make the diagnosis.

Ulna

Fracture of the olecranon can occur at any age, and it rarely represents a diagnostic problem. The olecranon ossification center should not be mistaken for a fracture in adolescents.

Fracture of the coronoid process is relatively uncommon and is difficult to visualize on either the AP or lateral projection because of the superimposition of other structures. Oblique views

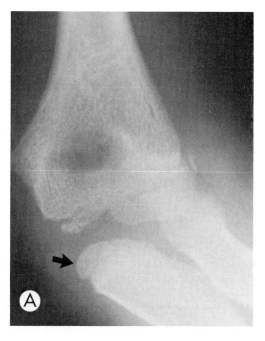
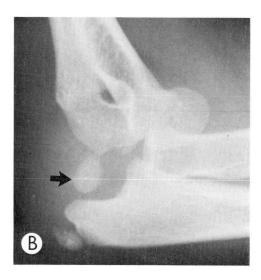

Fig. 9.   Dislocation of the elbow with avulsion and entrapment of the medial epicondylar ossification center in a 13-year-old child: (A) AP view. Note absence of the medial epicondylar ossification center from its usual position. It lies within joint (arrow) beneath the trochlear ossification center. (B) Lateral view demonstrates posterior displacement of the radius and ulna. Note the position of the medial epicondylar ossification center (arrow).

are necessary (Fig. 2). The fracture is created either by avulsion of the attached brachialis tendon or by impaction against the trochlea with or without an associated elbow dislocation. In either event, the line of fracture is located within 1 cm of the tip and is oriented in the coronal plane.

A fracture or dislocation of one of paired bones is almost always associated with a fracture or dislocation of the other. *Monteggia fracture* is a fracture of the proximal ulnar shaft associated with a dislocation of the proximal radius (Fig. 3).[8,10,15] It may occur at any age and is the result of a fall on the dorsal surface of the forearm. The fracture of the ulnar shaft is angulated anteriorly, and the proximal radius is dislocated anteriorly as well. Lateral or dorsal angulation and dislocation are rare. In young children the ulnar fracture may be incomplete, either of the greenstick variety or of the bowed type without a distinct line of fracture.[3] The most important aspect of the Monteggia fracture-dislocation is that the dislocation component is frequently overlooked[8] (Fig. 3).

Dislocation

Elbow dislocations are common. The radius and ulna are almost always posteriorly and laterally displaced. Occasionally, in adults, either the coronoid process of the ulna or the radial head is fractured as the ulna and radius are displaced posteriorly during the dislocation.[6] In children and adolescents, the medial epicondylar ossification center is frequently avulsed and may become entrapped during reduction (Fig. 9). The position of this center must be determined on both prereduction and postreduction radiographs.[5]

Isolated dislocation of one of paired bones is rarely encountered without an associated fracture or dislocation of the other bone, except in the case of *congenital dislocation of the radial head*. This can be identified readily by the rounded bulbous deformity of the radial head, lacking its normal shallow articular depression.

In infants and young children, the rare *separation of the entire distal humeral epiphysis*[17] may be confused with elbow dislocation. The diagnosis rests with the recognition that the radius and ulna are medially displaced, not laterally, as is characteristic of a dislocation (Fig. 10). The normal relationship of the capitellum and radius remains undisturbed, and therefore the distal humeral epiphysis must be displaced with the bones of the forearm.

The *jerked elbow* or *nursemaid elbow* occurs

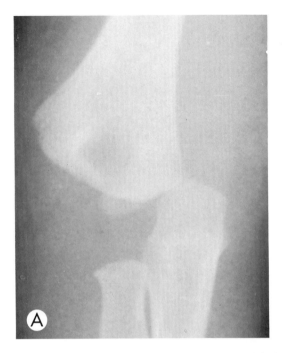

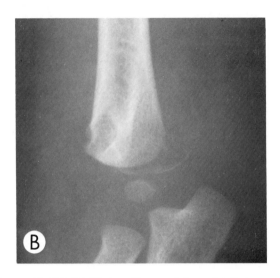

Fig. 10.   Separation of the entire distal humeral epiphysis in a 2-year-old child: (A) AP view. Characteristic medial displacement of the bones of the forearm. Note that the normal relationship of the radius to the capitellum has remained intact. (B) Oblique view. A metaphyseal fragment is evident. This is therefore a Salter type 2 injury.

in toddlers as a result of a sudden pull on the hand by an impatient adult.[15,18,21] The child begins to cry immediately and holds the forearm in midpronation. The exact anatomic abnormality is unknown. The roentgenographic examination is normal. The condition is cured by simply supinating the forearm. This may be accomplished by the x-ray technologist while positioning the forearm for the AP roentgenogram. Supination results in immediate relief of symptoms; the child ceases to cry, and the problem is solved.

REFERENCES

1. Bledsoe RC, Izenstark JL: Displacement of fat pads in disease and injury of the elbow: A new radiographic sign. Radiology 73:717–724, 1959

2. Bohrer SP: The fat pad sign following elbow trauma. Its usefulness and reliability in suspecting "invisible" fractures. Clin Radiol 21:90–94, 1970

3. Borden IVS: Roentgen recognition of acute plastic bowing of the forearm in children. Am J Roentgenol 125:524–530, 1975

4. Brogdon BG, Crow NE: Little leaguer's elbow. Am J Roentgenol 83:671–675, 1960

5. Chessare J, Rogers LF, Tachdjian MO, et al: Injuries of the medial epicondylar ossification center of the humerus. Am J Roentgenol 129:49–55, 1977

6. Eppright RH, Wilkins KE: Fractures and dislocations of the elbow, in Rockwood CA Jr, Green DP (eds): Fractures, vol. 1. Philadelphia, JB Lippincott, 1975, p 487

7. Flynn JC, Richards JF Jr: Non-union of minimally displaced fractures of the lateral condyle of the humerus in children. J Bone Joint Surg [Am] 53:1096–1101, 1971

8. Giustra PE, Killoran PJ, Furman RS, et al: The missed Monteggia fracture. Radiology 110:45–47, 1974

9. Hardacre JA, Nahigian SH, Froimson AI, et al: Fractures of the lateral condyle of the humerus in children. J Bone Joint Surg [Am] 53:1083–1095, 1971

10. Harris JH Jr, Harris WH: The radiology of emergency medicine (ed 1). Baltimore, Williams & Wilkins, 1975, p 139

11. Jeffery CC: Fractures of the neck of the radius in children. Mechanism of causation. J Bone Joint Surg [Br] 54:717–719, 1972

12. Kohn AM: Soft tissue alterations in elbow trauma. Am J Roentgenol 82:867–874, 1959

13. Nelson SW: Some important diagnostic and technical fundamentals in the radiology of trauma, with particular emphasis on skeletal trauma. Radiol Clin North Am 4:241–259, 1966

14. Norell HG: Roentgenologic visualization of the extracapsular fat, its importance in the diagnosis of traumatic injuries to the elbow. Acta Radiol 42:205–210, 1954

15. Rang M: Children's Fractures (ed 1). Philadelphia, Lippincott, 1974, p 93

16. Rogers LF: The radiography of epiphyseal injuries. Radiology 96:289–299, 1970

17. Rogers LF, Rockwood CA Jr: Separation of the entire distal humeral epiphysis. Radiology 106:393–400, 1973

18. Salter RB, Zaltz C: Anatomic investigations of the mechanism of injury and pathologic anatomy of "pulled elbow" in young children. Clin Orthop 77:134–143, 1971

19. Smith FM: Children's elbow injuries: Fractures and dislocations. Clin Orthop 50:7–30, 1967

20. Storen G: Traumatic dislocation of the radial head as an isolated lesion in children, report of one case with special regard to roentgen diagnosis. Acta Chir Scand 116:144–147, 1959

21. Tachdjian MO: Pediatric Orthopedics. Philadelphia, WB Saunders, 1972

22. Wadsworth TG: Injuries of the capitular (lateral humeral condylar) epiphysis. Clin Orthop 85:127–142, 1972

Hand and Wrist

Jeremy J. Kaye

ALTHOUGH fractures and dislocations in the hand and wrist are common, correct roentgenographic diagnosis may pose difficulty. Moreover, since these fractures involve small nonweight-bearing bones, there is a tendency to regard them as unimportant. Nothing could be further from the truth, for nowhere in the appendicular skeleton are structure and function so closely related. Thus it is important for the radiologist and his surgical colleagues to recognize shortening, angulation, and rotation of fracture fragments and to appreciate the potential for bony block of flexion or extension that may result during healing. In the carpus, the tendency toward instability following a dislocation can also significantly affect the functional ability of the upper extremity.

Intraarticular fractures are common in the hand and wrist, and an articular component should be carefully searched for, as it usually results in protracted pain and stiffness. If the articular surface is incongruous, there may be early onset of degenerative joint disease.

It is not possible here to describe all the types of fracture and dislocation that can occur in the hand and wrist. Rather, our concern will be with those that are important and those that are difficult to detect roentgenographically. The radiologist should realize that many significant injuries in the hand and wrist are not accompanied by fracture. Indeed, since their detection is more difficult, these soft-tissue injuries may be potentially more serious.

It is important for the radiologist to understand that his contribution to patient care does not end with initial diagnosis. He should be aware of possible complications and difficulties in treatment and should be careful and descriptive in the interpretation of follow-up radiographs.

PHALANGES

Distal Phalanx

Terminal tuft fracture is probably the most commonly encountered phalangeal fracture.[1] It may be exceedingly painful and may require evacuation of a subungual hematoma. Diagnosis is usually not difficult. Probably because of the many fibrous septa in the finger pulp, the fracture usually is not displaced, and complications are rare. Treatment is directed toward protection from further injury.

So-called baseball finger is another injury of the distal phalanx; it is also called mallet finger or dropped finger.[13] It results from a flexion force on the forcibly extended finger. Although it may be purely tendinous in origin, there may be an associated intraarticular fracture along the dorsum of the base of the phalanx (Figs. 1 and 2). Recognition of the characteristic deformity (flexion and volar subluxation at the distal interphalangeal joint) and the fracture fragment is the key to diagnosis. If the avulsed fragment of bone is large, surgical intervention may be necessary for complete functional recovery.

A functionally more important injury occurs on the volar aspect of the base of the distal phalanx, the *flexor digitorum profundus avulsion.*[2] It results from forced hyperextension of the flexed finger. It is usually a tendon injury, but there may be an intraarticular fracture. Roentgenographic detection, when no fracture is present, may require stress views with attempted finger flexion.

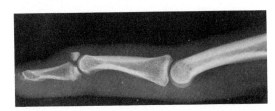

Fig. 1. "Baseball finger." There is an intraarticular fracture on the dorsum of the base of the distal phalanx. The proximal interphalangeal joint is in extension, while there is flexion and volar subluxation at the distal interphalangeal joint.

Jeremy J. Kaye, M.D.: *Associate Professor of Radiology, Department of Radiology, Associate Professor of Orthopedics and Rehabilitation, Vanderbilt University Hospital, Nashville, Tenn.*

Reprint requests should be addressed to Dr. Jeremy J. Kaye, Department of Radiology, Vanderbilt University Hospital, Nashville, Tenn. 37232.

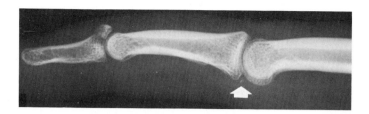

Fig. 2. Another "baseball finger," this time associated with intraarticular fracture of the distal insertion of the volar plate (arrow).

Middle and Proximal Phalanges

Intraarticular fractures are also important in this location. For return to normal function, involvement of the joint surfaces requires anatomic reduction, often needing surgical intervention with reduction and internal fixation. In these phalanges, muscle pull is often an important deforming force.

It is very important to recognize and treat rotational malalignment of fractures in these phalanges[11] (Fig. 3), although healing usually occurs without difficulty. Considerable functional impairment may result if rotation is not corrected, such as inability to clasp due to overlap of the fingers in flexion.

Volar plate injuries are quite common, and they may be difficult to detect roentgenographically.[11] Although they may be suspected on PA and oblique radiographs, they are often only clearly seen on the lateral view of the affected finger. These fractures, which are related to the insertion of the volar capsule and usually are due to hyperextension injuries, may be very small (Figs. 2 and 4). When the avulsed fracture fragment is large, open reduction and internal fixation may be necessary. A clue to the radiographic diagnosis may be hyperextension of the proximal interphalangeal joint. Some of the volar plate injuries also occur without a demonstrable fracture, and the hyperextension deformity may be the only roentgenographic clue.

The term *gamekeeper's thumb* refers to a disruption of the ulnar collateral ligament of the metacarpophalangeal joint of the thumb.[1,10] In wringing the necks of game, gamekeepers sustained chronic ligamentous injuries. The term is

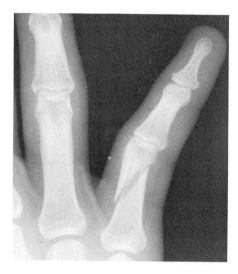

Fig. 3. Fracture of the proximal phalanx with rotational malalignment. While the ring finger is seen in PA projection, the distal portion of the little finger is seen obliquely.

currently applied to both chronic and acute injuries. In this country, the injury is often sustained from faulty handling of a ski pole.

Purely ligamentous injuries are not detectable on routine radiographs, and stress views are needed for diagnosis. Sometimes the injury is accompanied by a fracture of the base of the proximal phalanx (Fig. 5). Early diagnosis of complete ligamentous tears is important, as operative repair is often indicated. Failure to diagnose and treat this injury will result in diminished ability to pinch and to oppose the thumb.

METACARPALS

Metacarpal neck fractures are quite common. Perhaps the most frequently encountered

Fig. 4. Volar plate fracture with a very small avulsed fracture fragment (arrow).

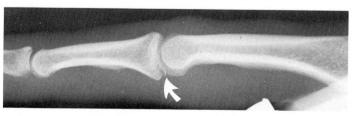

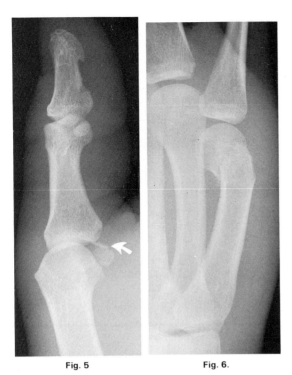

Fig. 5   Fig. 6.

Fig. 5.   Gamekeeper's thumb associated with a small intraarticular fracture near the insertion of the ulnar collateral
ligament (arrow).

Fig. 6.   Boxer's fracture of the fifth metacarpal head
with moderate dorsal angulation.

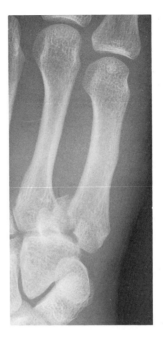

Fig. 7.   Fracture of the base of the fifth metacarpal with
intraarticular extension.

is the *boxer's fracture* of the fifth metacarpal
(Fig. 6). Angular deformity at the fracture site
is almost invariably noted. Since the volar
cortex is often comminuted, there is a tendency
for these fractures to settle backward after reduction, and careful note should be made of
such displacement.[11] Due to their greater mobility, fractures of the neck of the fourth and
fifth metacarpals are more sparing in terms of
permissible residual angulation. Residual loss of
function due to angulation is greater on the
radial side of the hand.

Metacarpal shaft fracture tends to angulate
dorsally due to the pull of the interosseous
muscles. If it is transverse, it is usually readily
reduced and held in position. However, oblique
fracture of the metacarpal shaft is often accompanied by both shortening and rotation. If
untreated, these may result in considerable impairment of function and position. The amount
of shortening and rotation should be carefully
noted on the initial and follow-up roentgenograms.

Fracture of the *metacarpal base* may also

have a rotational element that should be noted
and followed. An intraarticular component is
common, and it results in pain, stiffness, and
joint disease (Fig. 7); for this reason it may require operative intervention.

The thumb metacarpal deserves special men-
tion. Two related entities are the *Bennett fracture* and *Rolando fracture.* In the Bennett fracture, the thumb is fractured at the carpometa-

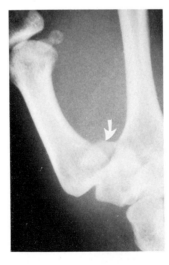

Fig. 8.   Bennett fracture of the base of the metacarpal of
the thumb. A small residual fragment (arrow) articulates
with the trapezium, while the remainder of the metacarpal is
dislocated.

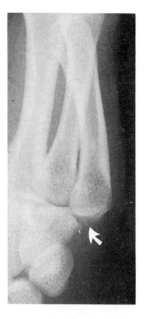

Fig. 9. Carpometacarpal fracture dislocation. Dorsal dislocation of the fifth metacarpal is noted on this oblique view, with a small chip fracture (arrow) of the dorsal surface of the hamate.

carpal joint; a small fragment of metacarpal continues to articulate with the trapezium, while the remainder of the metacarpal is dislocated (Fig. 8). A Rolando fracture is a comminuted Bennett fracture, with a separate dorsal fragment.

Other carpometacarpal dislocations occur, often accompanied by fractures.[17] These most commonly occur at the ulnar side of the wrist. Dislocation at the fourth or fifth carpometacarpal joint is not uncommon, and it may be accompanied by carpal fractures (Fig. 9). These dislocations are most commonly dorsal.

CARPUS

Scaphoid fractures are the most common type. These are often difficult to detect at the time of injury, and they may require special roentgenographic projections (Fig. 10). Frequently these fractures are radiographically undetectable at the time of injury and are recognized only on follow-up roentgenograms. A useful early sign is displacement of the navicular fat stripe.[14] Most of the complications from the injury are related to delay in diagnosis and institution of therapy. The most commonly encountered are delayed union, nonunion, and avascular necrosis. The more proximal the fracture line, the greater the likelihood of avascular necrosis.

Dorsal chip fractures occur without dislocation. The triquetrum is the most common site (Fig. 11). These are usually detected only on lateral or reverse oblique roentgenograms. They are usually uncomplicated.

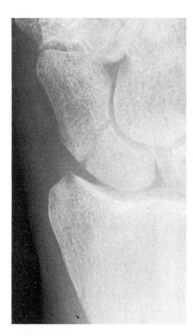

Fig. 10. Nondisplaced fracture of the scaphoid, visible only on this angled view in ulnar deviation.

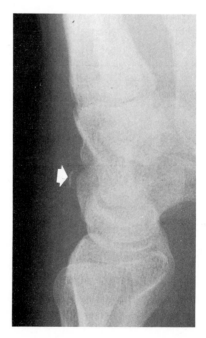

Fig. 11. Dorsal chip fracture of the triquetrium (arrow), visible only on the lateral radiograph.

Other carpal fractures are less common.[18] Supplemental radiographic projections may be necessary for diagnosis. In particular, fracture of the hook of the hamate is often best seen on the carpal tunnel projection and in the reverse oblique projection. The relatively common avascular necrosis of the lunate is probably secondary to a fracture.[11]

Dislocations

When a carpal fracture is detected, a careful check for the presence of an associated dislocation should also be made.[12,16,18] Carpal dislocations are ordinarily divided into lunate and perilunate types.[9,12,18] As pointed out by Linscheid et al[7] and by Rockwood and Green,[11] this is probably an artificial distinction. These authors have suggested the term *traumatic carpal instability* to include these entities, as well as carpal collapse patterns that may be secondary to such dislocations or sprains. They include scapholunar dissociation or rotatory dislocation (subluxation) of the scaphoid. The author agrees with this concept and has observed a number of cases that substantiate it.

The most common of the carpal dislocation patterns is the *transscaphoid perilunate dislocation* (Fig. 12). This consists of fracture of the waist of the navicular and dislocation (almost invariably dorsally) of the remainder of the carpus about the lunate and proximal pole of the navicular, which continue to remain in normal relationship to the distal radius. Fracture of the scaphoid implies that the scapholunar ligament is intact, although this is not invariably the case.

The pure *perilunate dislocation* occurs without a scaphoid fracture, and implies disruption of the scapholunar ligaments. Roentgenograms show a normal radiolunar relationship, with dislocation of the carpus, again almost invariably in the dorsal direction (Fig. 13). I have seen this type of dislocation progress, with or without treatment, to the classic lunate dislocation pattern. This type of dislocation may, after reduction, result in rotatory dislocation of the scaphoid or in a carpal collapse pattern.

Pure *lunate dislocation* may occur, but often it is secondary to perilunate dislocation. In lunate dislocation, the proximal articular surface of the lunate may be in partial contact with the distal radius, but its distal surface no longer

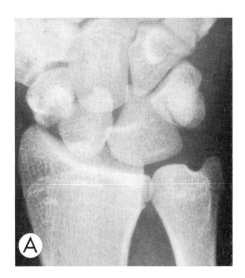

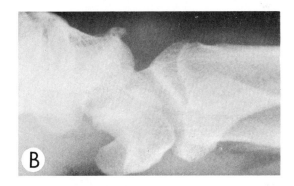

Fig. 12. Transscaphoid perilunate dislocation: (A) PA projection. The scaphoid fracture is readily demonstrable, as is the abnormal triangular configuration of the lunate. (B) Lateral projection shows the lunate in normal relationship with the distal radius and dorsal dislocation of the capitate and the remainder of the carpus. A small chip from the scaphoid fracture is evident dorsally.

articulates with the capitate (Fig. 14). As in the case of pure perilunate dislocation, a carpal collapse pattern, most frequently manifested by scapholunar dissociation, may ensue.

Rotatory subluxation of the scaphoid may occur without demonstrable prior dislocation. Many of these are diagnosed as wrist sprains.[6,15] The term *sprain* is nonspecific and implies that an injury is simple and that virtually all cases will have a good result. Nothing could be further from the truth, as premature onset of posttraumatic joint disease is a frequent complication. The roentgenographic clue in this instance is an abnormally wide distance between the navicular and the lunate (Fig. 15).

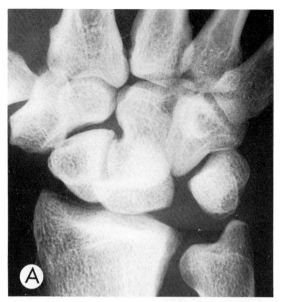

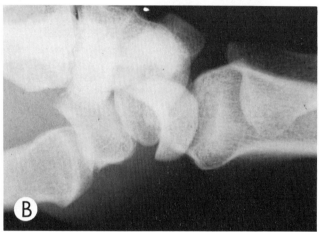

Fig. 13. Pure perilunate dislocation: (A) PA projection. No scaphoid fracture is evident. The abnormal triangular shape of the lunate is noted. (B) Lateral projection. The lunate is seen in normal relationship with the radius. The remainder of the carpus is dorsally dislocated.

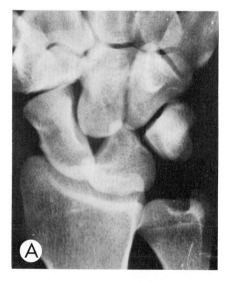

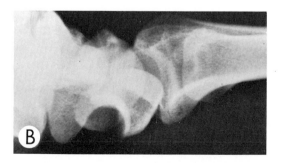

Fig. 14. Pure lunate dislocation: (A) PA projection reveals the abnormal triangular configuration of the lunate. (B) Lateral radiograph illustrates volar displacement of the lunate; its distal aspect no longer articulates with the capitate.

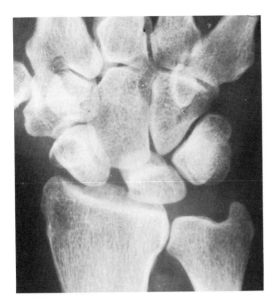

Fig. 15. Rotatory subluxation of the scaphoid or carpal collapse pattern. There is an abnormally wide distance between the scaphoid and the lunate.

DISTAL RADIUS AND ULNA

Fractures

Fractures of the distal radius and ulna are exceedingly common. Many of them have commonly used eponyms with which the radiologist should be familiar.

The most common of the fractures encountered is the *Colles fracture*. This is simply a distal radial fracture with dorsal displacement. It frequently is associated with a fracture of the ulnar styloid, although if there is no styloid fracture the eponym still applies. As with most fractures and dislocations in the upper extremity, the mechanism of injury is a fall on the outstretched hand. Most Colles fractures are

readily recognized on the lateral roentgenogram. A good roentgenographic clue to the diagnosis is an abnormal tilt to the distal radial articular surface (Fig. 16). Recall that there should normally be a volar tilt of the distal radial articular surface of approximately 15 degrees. There may be displacement of the fat pad over the pronator quadratus muscle.[8]

Many of these fractures have an intraarticular component, either into the radiocarpal joint or into the distal radioulnar joint. These extensions should be searched for, as they significantly affect prognosis; intraarticular fractures, particularly if displaced, frequently cause posttraumatic arthritis. In the follow-up period, careful attention should be paid to the radiocarpal angle, as these fractures tend to collapse. Shortening of the radius may result in dorsal dislocation of the ulna. Median nerve palsy may result, requiring a carpal tunnel release.

Smith fracture is a fracture of the distal radius with volar displacement of the distal fragment.[4] It is also referred to as a *reverse Colles fracture*. There may or may not be an intraarticular component. If one is present and the fracture line is oblique, maintenance of reduction is more difficult. A fracture with an intraarticular component is also referred to as *reverse Barton fracture*.

Fracture of the dorsal aspect of the radius may occur alone, and is referred to as *Barton fracture*. The carpus tends to sublux dorsally with the distal fragment of the radius, and the fracture is almost invariably intraarticular.[4]

Styloid fractures can occur in either the radius or the ulna. Fracture of the radial styloid is usually transverse and is best seen on the PA

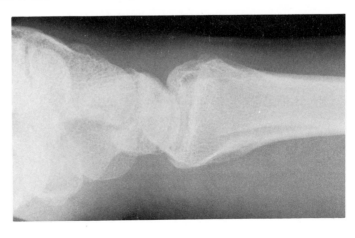

Fig. 16. Fracture of distal radius. This fracture, not recognized on other projections, was detected because of the abnormal dorsal tilt of the distal radial articular surface.

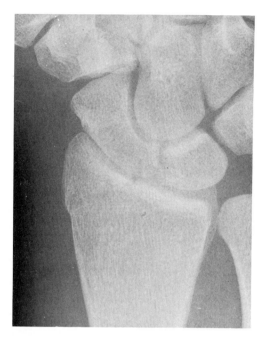

Fig. 17. Hutchinson or chauffeur's fracture, a transverse fracture of the radial styloid. It is best seen on the PA roentgenogram.

radiograph (Fig. 17). It is referred to as the *Hutchinson* or *chauffeur's fracture*. The latter name dates from the time of hand-cranked automobiles, when direct trauma to the radial side of the wrist could be sustained from the crank.

Ulnar styloid fracture is a common concomitant of other distal radial fractures, but it may be an isolated injury. This fracture is unimportant compared with the associated injury to the radius.

Dislocations

Distal radioulnar dislocations are almost invariably dorsal, and they can easily be overlooked, especially if the film has not been made in true lateral projection, as often happens in the acutely injured patient. In the absence of a styloid fracture, and even in the absence of ulnar dislocation, there may still be a significant injury at the distal radioulnar joint: tear of the triangular fibrocartilage. This can be detected by wrist arthrography.

Galeazzi fracture is a fracture of the distal third of the radius accompanied by dorsal dislocation of the ulna. This fracture is also called a *reverse Monteggia fracture.* In my experience, these are rare indeed.

REFERENCES

1. Campbell CS: Gamekeeper's thumb. J Bone Joint Surg [Br] 37:148–149, 1955
2. Carroll RE, Match RM: Avulsion of the flexor profundus tendon insertion. J Trauma 11:366–371, 1953
3. Dameron TB Jr: Traumatic dislocation of the distal radio-ulnar joint. Clin Orthop 83:55–63, 1972
4. Ellis J: Smith's and Barton's fractures. A method of treatment. J Bone Joint Surg [Br] 47:724–727, 1965
5. Head RW: Anterior dislocation of the distal ulna without accompanying fracture of the ulnar styloid. Br J Radiol 44:468-471, 1971
6. Hudson TM, Caragol WJ, Kaye JJ: Isolated rotatory subluxation of the carpal navicular. Am J Roentgenol 126:601–611, 1976
7. Linscheid RL, Dobyns JH, Beabout JW: Traumatic instability of the wrist: Diagnosis, classification, and pathomechanics. J Bone Joint Surg [Am] 54:1612–1632, 1972
8. MacEwan DW: Changes due to trauma in the fat plane overlying the pronator quadratus muscle. A radiologic sign. Radiology 82:879–886, 1964
9. Nelson SW: Some important diagnostic and technical fundamentals in the radiology of trauma, with particular emphasis on skeletal trauma. Radiol Clin North Am 4:241–259, 1966
10. Resnick D, Danzig LA: Arthrographic evaluation of injuries on the first metacarpophalangeal joint: Gamekeeper's thumb. Am J Roentgenol 126:1046–1052, 1976
11. Rockwood CA, Green DP: Fractures. Philadelphia, JB Lippincott, 1975
12. Russell TB: Inter-carpal dislocations and fracture dislocations: A review of fifty-nine cases. J Bone Joint Surg [Br] 31:524–531, 1949
13. Stark HH, Boyes JH, Wilson JN: Mallet finger. J Bone Joint Surg [Am] 44:1061–1068, 1962
14. Terry DW Jr, Ramin JE: The navicular fat stripe: A useful roentgen feature for evaluating wrist trauma. Am J Roentgenol 124:25–28, 1975
15. Thompson TC, Campbell RD Jr, Arnold WD: Primary and secondary dislocation of the scaphoid bone. J Bone Joint Surg [Br] 46:73–82, 1964
16. Wagner CJ: Fracture dislocations of the wrist. Clin Orthop 15:181-196 1959
17. Waugh RL, Yancey AG: Carpometacarpal dislocations: With particular reference to simultaneous dislocation of the bases of the fourth and fifth metacarpals. J Bone Joint Surg [Am] 30:397–404, 1948
18. Wiot JF, Dorst JP: Less common fractures and dislocations of the wrist. Radiol Clin North Am 4:261–276, 1966

Bony Pelvis and Hip

Alvin Thaggard III, Thomas S. Harle, and Victor Carlson

FRACTURES OF THE PELVIS

Fractures of the pelvis, while comprising only a low percentage of all skeletal fractures, are extremely important because of their significant morbidity and mortality (4%–19%).[14,58] Hemorrhage requiring transfusion occurs in 20%–40% of these patients,[58,60] and hemorrhagic shock and its complications are the major causes of death.[9,29,52] Associated soft-tissue damage often is more important than the fracture. Injury of the lower urinary tract is so frequent that it should be considered to be present until proved otherwise.

Anatomy

The bony pelvic ring consists of two innominate bones and the sacrum, bound anteriorly by the strong interpubic ligaments and posteriorly by the sacroiliac ligaments. The large fan-shaped innominate bone is comprised of three separate bones: ilium, ischium, and pubis. In the second decade, the three fuse at the triradiate cartilage, forming the acetabulum. The rami of the ischium and pubis enclose the obturator foramen. We will refer to them jointly as the superior and inferior ischiopubic rami.

Two main arches form the major support of the pelvis, and each is stabilized by a subsidiary or tie arch. The more important femorosacral arch extends from one acetabulum to the other, containing the ilia, sacroiliac joints, and sacrum. This is augmented by a tie arch between the acetabula through the pubic bones. This complex forms what commonly is referred to as the bony pelvic ring. The less important ischiopubic arch forms the main support in the sitting position.

Since the bony pelvis is nearly a rigid ring, when one is confronted with an apparent single break, the pelvis should be carefully scrutinized for a second fracture of the ring or sacroiliac joint or pubic symphysis diastasis. However, due to the slight motion at these joints and the inherent elasticity of bone, solitary fracture of the ring does occur.

Roentgen Examination

An AP view is frequently the only roentgenogram obtained of the pelvis. Unfortunately, for full delineation of injury, the complex bony anatomy of this area often requires additional projections, such as oblique, lateral, AP with 35-degree cephalic tilt, and inlet (caudal tilt) views.

In addition to inspecting the bones, a search should be made for subtle soft-tissue signs of hemorrhage or urinary extravasation, such as elevation of small bowel loops, abnormal position of the bladder, and displacement or obliteration of the fat planes of the pelvis and lower abdomen.[25,61]

The urinary tract is frequently at risk in pelvic fractures. Bladder injury has been reported in 6% and urethral injury in nearly 10% of cases.[7,8] The urinary tract should be examined as soon as the patient's condition permits. An intravenous urogram allows evaluation of the kidneys and ureters, but it should not be relied on for evaluation of the bladder or urethra. Retrograde urethrography should precede blind insertion of a bladder catheter in most, if not all, patients with pelvic trauma. If normal, a high-volume (250–300 cc) cystogram should be performed through an indwelling catheter. Urethral rupture associated with pelvic fractures occurs almost exclusively in males and is seen with major diastasis of the symphysis pubis or fractures about the pubis. Bladder rupture, which is less common, may

Alvin Thaggard III, M.D.: *Assistant Professor of Radiology, Department of Radiology, The University of Texas Medical School at Houston, Hermann Hospital, Houston, Texas.* Thomas S. Harle, M.D.: *Professor and Chairman, Department of Radiology, The University of Texas Medical School at Houston, Hermann Hospital, Houston, Texas.* Victor Carlson, M.D.: *Assistant Clinical Professor of Diagnostic Radiology, Department of Radiology, St. Joseph's Hospital, Houston, Texas.*

Reprint requests should be addressed to Apt. 209, Rosa Verde Towers, 343 West Houston, San Antonio, Texas 78205.

© 1978 by Grune & Stratton, Inc.

0037-198X/78/1302-0006$0200/0

Table 1

I. Stable pelvic fractures (67%)[33]
   A. Avulsion fracture
   B. Iliac wing fracture
   C. Sacral fracture
   D. Fracture of the ischiopublic Rami
II. Unstable pelvic fractures (33%): two or more fractures and/or diastases in the bony ring
   A. Straddle fracture (comminuted fracture of tie arch)
   B. Double vertical fracture and/or dislocation
      1. Malgaigne fracture (ipsilateral)
      2. Pelvic dislocation
      3. Bucket-handle fracture (contralateral)
   C. Total pelvic disruption

result from the piercing action of a bony spicule or from compressive forces, especially on a full bladder.[8] Water-soluble contrast enema may be indicated in patients with signs of colonic or rectal injury.

Pelvic arteriography and venography may be extremely valuable for both diagnosis and therapy of vascular injury and hemorrhage.[2,24,40,57,59] Surgical control of massive pelvic bleeding has been notoriously difficult.[19] Transfemoral arteriography may localize the bleeding site, which can then be treated with balloon catheter, embolic vascular occlusion with autologous clot, or synthetic material such as Gelfoam.[6,40,59] Major vascular injury such as arterial occlusion, intimal damage, pseudoaneurysm, or arteriovenous fistula may also be detected.[5,31,59,69] Transfemoral venography may demonstrate laceration of the iliac veins, a common cause of excessive hemorrhage,[46] and should follow arteriography if no bleeding site is

identified or if there is continued hemorrhage following arterial embolization.[59]

To emphasize the stability of the injury, we have adopted a modification of the classifications of Dunn and Morris[14] and Pennal and Sutherland[54] (Table 1). Acetabular fractures, due to involvement of a major weight-bearing joint, will be considered separately.

Stable Pelvic Fractures

Avulsion Fractures

Avulsion fractures most commonly occur in athletes, prior to fusion of the involved apophyseal center, from forcible muscular contraction (Fig. 1). The anterior superior iliac spine, which unites with the ilium at about 16 to 20 years of age, is avulsed by the sartorius muscle, particularly in sprinters. Avulsion of the anterior inferior iliac spine occurs less commonly and is caused by contraction of the rectus femoris. The latter should not be confused with an ununited os acetabuli. The ossification center of the ischial tuberosity, which often does not fuse until age 25, may be avulsed by contraction of the hamstring complex, an injury seen in hurdlers and cheerleaders.

In healing, exuberant callus may form, producing an appearance that has been confused with neoplasm.[4,16,28,70] Avulsion injuries near the symphysis pubis, caused by pull of the adductor muscle complex, have been described recently in young athletes, and may simulate infection or neoplasm radiographically.[65] Treat-

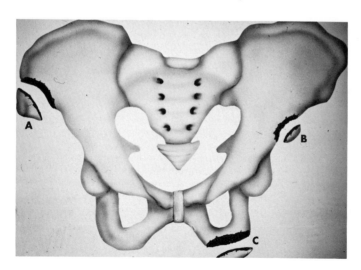

Fig. 1. Avulsion fractures: (A) anterior superior iliac spine; (B) anterior inferior iliac spine; (C) ischial tuberosity. (Reproduced by permission from Dunn and Morris.[14])

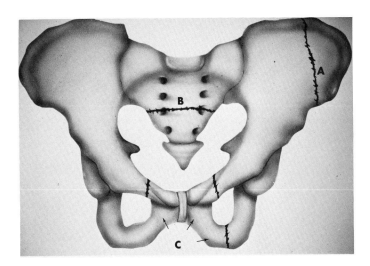

Fig. 2. Stable fractures of the pelvic ring: (A) iliac wing; (B) body of sacrum; (C) pubic rami. (Reproduced by permission from Dunn and Morris.[14])

ment of these fractures is usually nonsurgical.[28,60]

Iliac Wing Fracture

The iliac wing fracture, first reported by Duverney,[15] usually is caused by direct force from a lateral direction, often displacing the iliac wing medially but not involving the pelvic ring per se (Fig. 2). Oblique views are of greater diagnostic value than the AP view in most cases.

Fractures of the Sacrum

Sacral fractures are of two major varieties: (1) Those caused by direct trauma, such as a fall in the sitting position, are most often horizontal and occasionally are displaced. They are best visualized on the lateral view (Fig. 2); the AP view may appear perfectly normal. (2) Those caused by indirect trauma, such as a blow to the pelvis, knee, or foot, often result in a vertical fracture, which represents a break in the pelvic ring (Fig. 3)[44].

The incidence of sacral fracture associated with another pelvic fracture has been variously reported from 4% to 74% of patients.[20,76] This wide discrepancy may reflect the frequency with which the vertical fracture is overlooked. It commonly is visible in the AP but not the lateral

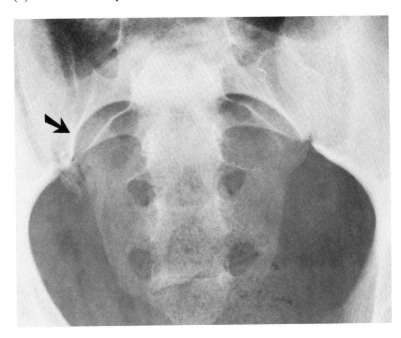

Fig. 3. Vertical sacral fracture. Commonly overlooked, this injury frequently accompanies fracture of the pelvic ring at another location, and it is best seen in the frontal projection. There is a torus-type fracture of the anterior superior sacral foraminal line (arrow) and a radiolucent vertical component below this site.

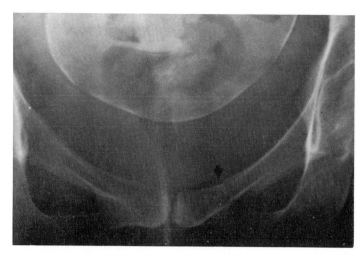

Fig. 4. Stress fracture (arrow) of superior pubic ramus in late pregnancy.

view and is manifested by a discontinuity or asymmetry of one or more of the anterior superior sacral foramina lines. One or more of the lines may merely show buckling, similar to a torus fracture of an extremity (Fig. 3). It has also been reported as an isolated injury.[51] The AP cephalic tilt view or tomography may be necessary for diagnosis.

Fractures of Ischiopubic Rami

Fractures involving the ischiopubic rami are the most common fractures of the pelvis (Fig. 2).[33,56] The stability of these injuries results from the inherent strength of the obturator ring. As a result of the posterior slope of the pubis, the fractures are often better visualized on a 35-degree cephalic tilt view, which may also be the best frontal view for the sacrum. An inlet view, taken with 15 to 30 degrees of caudal tilt, may show displacement of fracture fragments more clearly. Treatment is usually symptomatic.[60]

Stress fractures of the rami are occasionally seen in the third trimester of pregnancy (Fig. 4),[34] in military recruits after prolonged marching,[66] and in osteopenia of various causes.[71]

Unstable Pelvic Fractures

Straddle Fractures

The straddle fracture or comminuted fracture of the tie arch is the most common type of unstable fracture.[9,14,53] The classic appearance is that of bilateral fractures of all four ischiopubic rami (Fig. 5), although ipsilateral ischiopubic ramus fractures and separation of

the symphysis pubis may occur. Bladder rupture and urethral tear occur in about one-third of patients.[9] Despite their classification as unstable, treatment of these fractures is largely symptomatic.[60]

Double Vertical Fracture/Dislocation

The pelvic ring, both anterior and posterior to the acetabulum, is involved. This is a more significant injury than the straddle fracture, since treatment must be aimed at reduction of fracture fragments as well as at the commonly associated visceral injury. Three major types exist:

Malgaigne fracture. The Malgaigne fracture,[39] by far the most common of the three, involves one hemipelvis. Most commonly, there are fractures of both ipsilateral ischiopubic rami or separation of the symphysis pubis, as well as fracture about or dislocation of the sacroiliac joint (Fig. 6). Superior or posterior displacement of the entire hemipelvis may occur, with fracture of the L-5 transverse process. The

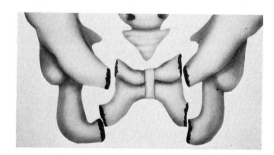

Fig. 5. Straddle fracture (comminuted fracture of the arch). (Reproduced by permission from Dunn and Morris.[14])

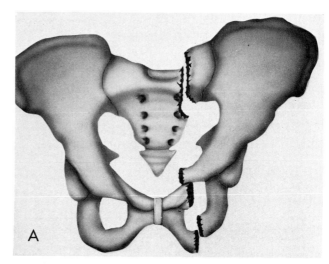

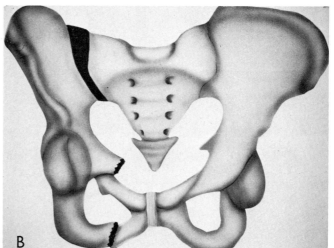

Fig. 6. Malgaigne fracture: (A) with ipsilateral double vertical fractures; (B) with dislocation of sacroiliac joint as the posterior component. (Reproduced by permission from Dunn and Morris.[14])

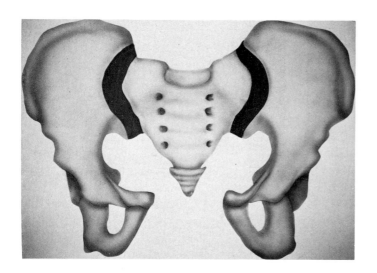

Fig. 7. Pelvic dislocation or "sprung pelvis" (Reproduced by permission from Dunn and Morris.[14])

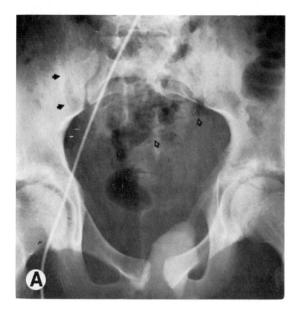
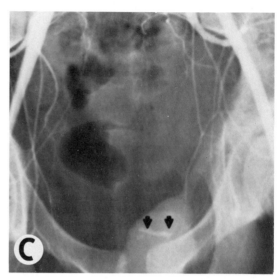
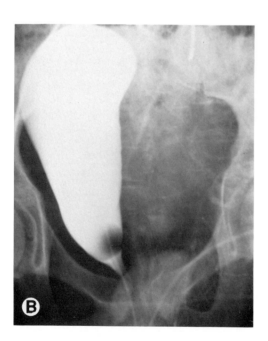
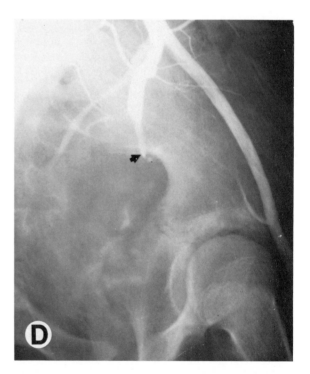

Fig. 8. Pelvic dislocation from an auto accident in a 14-year-old boy in hypovolemic shock: (A) AP pelvis showing pubic diastasis, dislocation of right sacroiliac joint (closed arrows), and elevation of bowel loops (open arrows) from pelvic hematoma. (B) Cystogram, demonstrating a large pelvic hematoma. (C) Aortogram on day of injury, showing active arterial bleeding site (arrows). The attending physicians decided to watch the patient, but following 14 units of blood in 12 hours angiographic embolization was requested. (D) Left iliac arteriography following Gelfoam embolization of the internal iliac artery (arrow) demonstrates complete occlusion and cessation of hemorrhage. The patient tolerated the embolization well and did not require exploratory surgery.

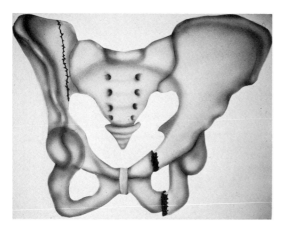

Fig. 9. Bucket-handle or contralateral double vertical fracture. (Reproduced by permission from Dunn and Morris.[14])

mode of injury may be direct or indirect compression.[13] This fracture involves high morbidity and mortality[9,32] and may be complicated by rupture of the diaphragm.

Pelvic dislocation. Pelvic dislocation or "sprung pelvis" is a related injury (Figs. 7 and 8). There is separation of the symphysis pubis and one or both sacroiliac joints caused by anterior compressive forces.[14] Normally the distance between the pubic bones should not exceed 8 mm in nonpregnant adults or 10 mm in children.[48] The superior margins of the pubic bones may normally be aligned on slightly different planes, but the inferior borders have been found to lie in the same plane in 99.5% of normal males and 95% of normal females.[74] Therefore the sacrum and sacroiliac joints should be carefully inspected in any trauma case with slight asymmetry of the inferior pubic borders. Again, hemorrhage and lower urinary tract injury are common, since the urogenital diaphragm containing the posterior urethra is disrupted.

Bucket-handle fracture. The bucket-handle fracture or contralateral double vertical fracture (Fig. 9) is due to oblique forces and involves both ischiopubic rami on the side opposite the impact, combined with fracture about or dislocation of the sacroiliac joint on the side of impact. The hemipelvis may be rotated and displaced upward and inward. Although retroperitoneal hemorrhage is common, urinary tract damage is reported to be rare.[14]

Total Pelvic Disruption

The comminuted crush fracture of total pelvic disruption involves three or more of the components of the pelvic ring and carries the highest morbidity and mortality of all pelvic fractures.[73]

HIP JOINT INJURIES

Fractures of the Acetabulum

The innominate bone may be considered to have two columns of bone forming a 60-degree angle: a posterior ilioischial column and an anterior iliopubic column. The acetabulum is bordered by the thick condyloid labrum, incomplete only inferiorly. The broad quadrilateral

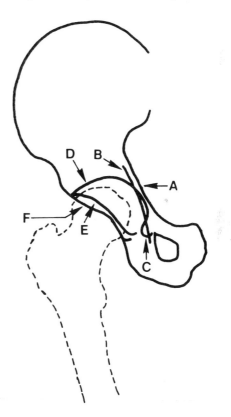

Fig. 10. The six lines of the acetabulum seen in AP projection: A, the iliopubic line extending from the greater sciatic notch to the pubic tubercle; B, the ilioischial line formed by the posterior portion of the quadrilateral plate; C, the teardrop or roentgen U formed laterally by the medial acetabular wall, inferiorly by the acetabular notch, and medially by the anterior portion of the quadrilateral plate. In a true AP view the ilioischial line should cross or lie tangential to the teardrop; D, roof of the acetabulum; E, anterior lip; F, posterior lip. (Reproduced by permission from Judet et al.[37])

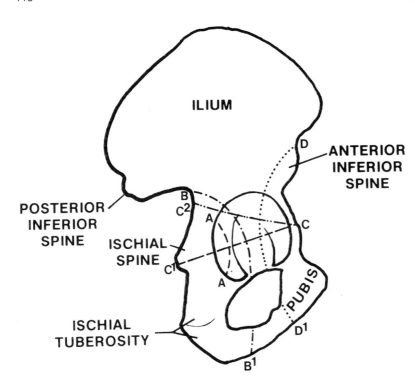

Fig. 11. Basic fractures of the acetabulum shown on a lateral view of the innominate bone. A-A^1, posterior rim fracture; B-B^1, posterior (ilioischial) column fracture; C-C^1, central transverse fracture; C-C^2, central oblique fracture; D-D^1, anterior (iliopubic) column fracture.

plate on the medial surface of the innominate bone forms the inner wall of the acetabulum.

In the AP projection, six bony landmarks should be identified (Fig. 10).[37] In suspected acetabular injury, at least four views should be obtained when the patient's condition warrants: (1) AP hip; (2) AP pelvis (because of the frequency of bilateral injuries); (3) 45-degree external oblique, which shows the posterior column and anterior lip; (4) 45-degree internal oblique, which shows the anterior column and posterior lip. Tomography, groin lateral, and supine cross-table lateral views may be of value.[45]

The fat plane overlying the thin origin of the obturator internus muscle from the quadrilateral plate should be observed for displacement or asymmetry, the positive obturator internus sign (Fig. 13A). This is a sensitive indicator of hematoma beneath or within this muscle.

Almost all acetabular fractures are due to indirect trauma, via force to the foot, knee, or greater femoral trochanter. This type of fracture is related most commonly to the position of the femur at the time of impact. According to the classification of Judet et al,[37] four basic fractures exist (Fig. 11).

Posterior Rim Fracture

The posterior rim or dashboard fracture usually occurs after a blow to the knee with the leg in flexion and adduction. The commonly associated posterior dislocation of the hip, as well as the fracture itself, may be subtle on the AP view (Fig. 12).

Simple Posterior Column Fracture

The simple posterior column fracture is uncommon. On the AP view, the ilioischial line is displaced medially and separated from the tear-drop. It is best seen on the external oblique projection.

Central Acetabular Fracture

The central acetabular fracture is the most common acetabular fracture. It divides the innominate bone into superior and inferior halves. In the transverse type, the fracture line bisects the ischial spine (Fig. 13). The oblique type extends posterosuperiorly through the quadrilateral plate toward the sacrosciatic notch (Fig. 14). The oblique fracture may be extremely difficult to diagnose due to the anteroposterior orientation of the quadrilateral plate. A positive obturator internus sign may be the only finding

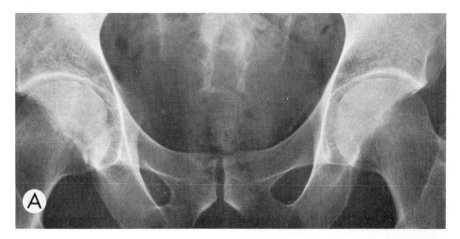

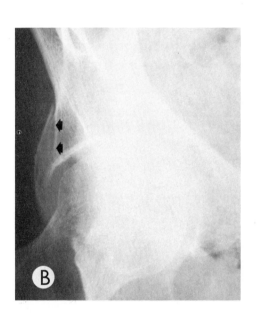

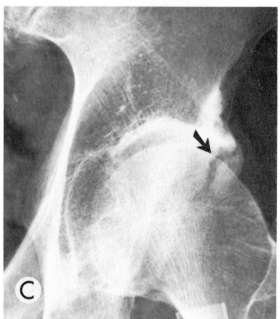

Fig. 12. Posterior acetabular rim fracture: (A) AP pelvis. The fracture is not well seen. (B) Posterior oblique view of right hip clearly demonstrates the fracture (arrow). (C) Another patient. The unfused os acetabuli (arrow) should not be confused with a fracture.

on the AP view,[61] and oblique views or tomography are often necessary for diagnosis. If the fracture is severe, there may be central dislocation of the femoral head (Fig. 15).

Simple Anterior Column Fracture

The simple anterior column fracture may terminate inferiorly in various locations along the pubis or ischiopubic junction. On the AP view there is loss of continuity of the iliopubic line and medial displacement of the teardrop

with respect to the ilioischial line (Fig. 16). The internal oblique is the view of choice.

These four basic fractures accounted for nearly two-thirds of the acetabular fractures in the series of Judet et al, with combinations or variations comprising the remainder.

Rowe and Lowell[62] proposed a different classification, emphasizing the importance of the condition of the superior weight-bearing dome, as well as the condition of the femoral head, the adequacy of the reduction, and the stability of the joint after reduction.

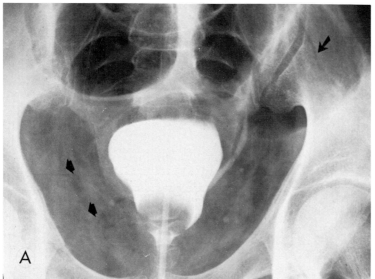

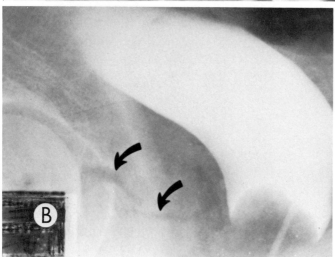

Fig. 13. Low central acetabular fracture on the right: (A) AP urogram. A large pelvic hematoma has displaced the bladder. There is a positive obturator internus sign (arrowheads). A fracture of the left ilium (arrow) is also present. (B) The posterior oblique view demonstrates the fracture extending medially to the ischial spine (arrows).

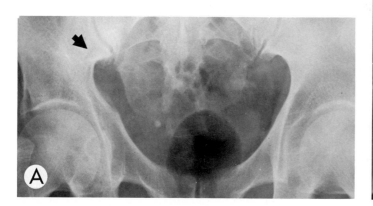

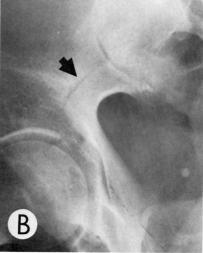

Fig. 14. Oblique central acetabular fracture: (A) AP pelvis, showing slight irregularity of the iliopubic line and a subtle fracture line (arrow) near the right sacrosciatic notch (arrow). (B) This is better seen on the posterior oblique view.

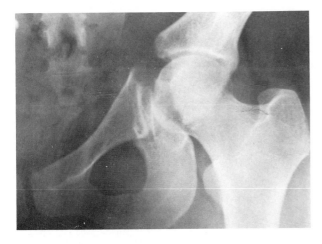

Fig. 15. Central fracture dislocation of the left hip.

Often, specific classification of the injury is difficult; in some cases it is unimportant. However, it is important to observe the "six lines" of the acetabulum and to know that commonly subtle central fractures are visualized only on the oblique view and manifest on the AP film merely by a positive obturator internus sign, and that there is a common association between acetabular fracture and fracture of the inferior ischiopubic ramus.

Dislocation of the Hip

The ball-and-socket hip joint is supported mainly by the iliofemoral, iliopubic, and ischiofemoral ligaments, which enclose the femoral head in a capsule. Dislocations may be classified as anterior, posterior, or central, any

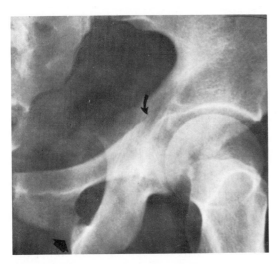

Fig. 16. Simple fracture of the anterior column. AP of left hip demonstrating loss of continuity of the iliopubic line (curved arrow) and fracture of the ischiopubic junction (arrow).

of which may be associated with fracture of the acetabulum or femoral head.

Anterior Dislocation

Anterior dislocation accounts for only 13% of dislocations.[18] It is caused by forced abduction and usually extension of the femur. The final position of the femoral head, ie, in the obturator, pubic, or iliac region, depends on the position of the femur at the time of injury. The roentgen picture is that of abduction, external rotation, and either flexion (obturator type) or extension (iliac or pubic type). The femoral head is commonly medial and inferior to the acetabulum on the AP view (Fig. 17). Associated fractures of the femoral head or acetabular rim may not be appreciated until a postreduction film is made.

Posterior Dislocation

Posterior dislocation is the most common type, and it occurs following a blow to the foot or knee with the hip in flexion. Abduction of the thigh at the time of injury may result also in a fracture of the posterior lip of the acetabulum. Roentgenographically, the femur is usually in internal rotation, flexion, and adduction, and the femoral head lies lateral and superior to the acetabulum on the AP view (Figs. 17 and 18). The dislocation is not always obvious on the AP view[47,77] (Fig. 19). However, loss of continuity in Shenton line or discrepancy in femoral head size may be a clue. Oblique, groin-lateral, stereoscopic views or even tomography may frequently be necessary for the complete diagnosis of the dislocation and associated fractures.

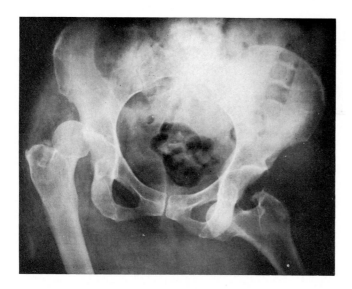

Fig. 17. Bilateral dislocation of the hips. The AP film of the pelvis shows a typical posterior dislocation of the right hip with adduction, flexion, and internal rotation of femur. On the left, there is a typical obturator type of anterior dislocation. There were no associated fractures.

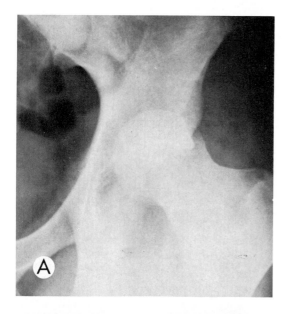

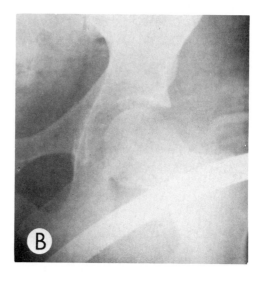

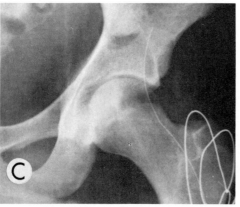

Fig. 18. Posterior fracture-dislocation of the left hip: (A) AP view before reduction. (B) AP view post reduction, demonstrating medial and superior widening of the joint space indicating possible interposed fragment. The patient remained symptomatic and had limited range of motion. (C) AP view of pelvis following surgical removal of interposed fragments, demonstrating a normal joint space.

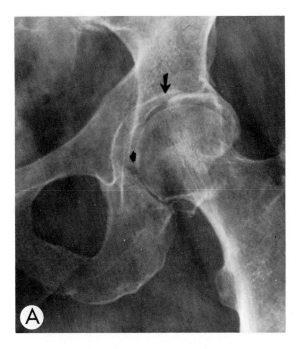

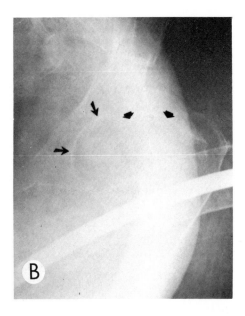

Fig. 19. Fracture-dislocation of the left femoral head: (A) AP view of hip demonstrating loss of continuity of the ilioischial line (arrowhead) and acetabular roof (arrow) plus subtle loss of the posterior acetabular rim shadow inferiorly. (B) The anterior oblique view shows complete dislocation of the femoral head (arrowheads) from the left acetabulum (arrows).

Asymmetry of the hip joint spaces of greater than 2 mm on a nonrotated postreduction film of the pelvis should suggest interposed osteochondral fragments, which may prevent adequate reduction and require surgical removal (Fig. 18). Tomography often is useful for demonstrating such fragments, as well as the subtle impacted fractures of the femoral head.[68]

With prompt reduction, the end result is satisfactory in the majority of cases. Epstein[17] and others advocate open reduction, when possible, in all cases of fracture dislocation, as they believe that fragments are always present in the joint.

Central Fracture/Dislocation

Central fracture/dislocation has been discussed with acetabular fractures (Fig. 15).

Complications

Aseptic necrosis of the femoral head may follow any type of dislocation. Its incidence becomes higher the longer reduction is delayed, approaching 50% at 24 hours in posterior dislocations.[60] It may appear as late as 2 years after injury. Post-traumatic arthrosis is occasionally seen, particularly when avascular necrosis is present or when an interposed fragment has remained in the joint. It is therefore less common after surgical reduction.[18] Myositis ossificans or capsular ossification is more common after open reduction.[60]

Sciatic nerve paralysis from pressure by the femoral head or a displaced acetabular fragment occurs in about 10% of cases of posterior dislocation.[35]

FRACTURES OF THE PROXIMAL FEMUR

Anatomy

In normal adults, the neck of the femur projects from the shaft at an angle of 120–130 degrees medially and 15–20 degrees anteriorly. The long axis of the medial femoral neck, containing important weight-bearing trabeculae, forms an angle of about 160 degrees with the long axis of the shaft in the AP view (Garden angle,[21,22] and 180 degrees in the lateral view.

The articular capsule of the hip is attached around the acetabular rim proximally and along a line roughly paralleling the intertrochanteric crest distally. A network of fibers extending from the inferior capsule reflects along the neck of the femur and thins out as it approaches the head of the femur. It makes up the retinaculum, binding the capsule closely to the femoral neck.

The major blood supply of the femoral head arises from branches of the medial and lateral femoral circumflex arteries, which form a vascular ring around the femoral neck. The branches pass under the capsule and are at risk in intracapsular fracture or dislocation of the hip. The only other significant blood supply to the head of the femur is a small, sometimes rudimentary, group of vessels in the ligamentum teres that may become important in revascularizing an ischemic femoral head.

Incidence

Fractures of the proximal femur occur most commonly in the elderly, often with only minor trauma. Of course, pathologic changes in this area, such as malignancy, radiation necrosis, and metabolic bone diseases such as osteoporosis, osteomalacia, and Paget disease, predispose to fracture. Fracture of the femur is rare in Negroes[27] and is said to be rare in the osteoarthritic hip.[41] Indices of osteoporosis have been used to predict the occurrence of hip fracture.[49,50,75]

The overall incidence in females is twice that in males, but it is five times that in males when considering intracapsular fractures alone.[3] The average age is around 70 years; extracapsular fractures occur in a slightly older population.

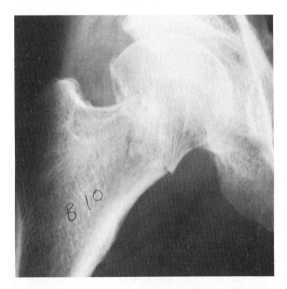

Fig. 20. Impacted fracture of the right femoral neck. A valgus deformity is associated with the impaction. AP view.

Roentgen Examination

Right angle views are important but often difficult to obtain. The lateral view of choice is the groin-lateral, taken with horizontal beam and grid cassette. No motion of the involved hip is required, and this projection best demonstrates the angulation and comminution of femoral neck fractures. The lateral view, a coned AP view, and an AP pelvis should constitute the initial examination.

Classification

From a clinical standpoint, these fractures are best divided into intracapsular and extracapsular types, as there is variation in the treatment and prognosis of the two. While almost all extracapsular fractures are due to a fall, there is a question whether a fall on the hip results from or leads to some intracapsular injuries.[21,26,36,43]

Intracapsular Fracture

Fracture of the femoral head is often associated with dislocation of the hip, and it may be difficult to diagnose on a single film. Stress and impacted fractures of the femoral neck often present a diagnostic dilemma both clinically and radiographically. Careful inspection of the medial femoral neck and head, the normal trabecular lines, length of the femoral neck, and Shenton line is mandatory. Occasionally the only roentgen sign of an impacted fracture is a linear area of increased density in the femoral neck. In undisplaced femoral neck fractures, the fracture line is remarkably constant, forming about a 55-degree angle with the long axis of the femur.[38] The upper limit of the fracture commences at the epiphyseal scar and descends through the neck of the femur to include a spike of dense medial cortical bone of varying length (Fig. 20). In displaced fractures of the femoral neck, the distal fragment is usually in external rotation, medial angulation, and cephalic displacement. Comminution of the posterior neck is a common feature.[22,23,64] Prompt surgery is indicated in displaced fractures to avoid further complications.[60]

Extracapsular Fracture of the Hip

This group includes those fractures occurring along the base of the neck of the femur just above the trochanteric line, through the trochanteric region, and distally to a level just below the trochanteric line, sometimes including a varying length of the proximal femoral shaft. Occasionally differentiation between intracapsular and extracapsular fractures is not possible. Detailed classifications of extracapsular fractures have been proposed, based on the type of reduction and fixation required,[72] but a more important issue is whether the fracture is stable or unstable. The stable fracture may be simple or minimally comminuted, with small, slightly separated, greater or lesser trochanteric fragments. The posterior wall of the femur is not significantly disrupted. The unstable fracture, on the other hand, is one with significant comminution of the medial or posterior femoral cortex, often with a large posteromedial fragment that includes the lesser trochanter. The inferior beak of the proximal fragment may be wedged into the medullary cavity of the distal fragment or displaced medial to it, and the greater trochanter may be broken off and widely separated. This constitutes the so-called four-part fracture (Fig. 21).

All components of the extracapsular hip fracture must be recognized in order to achieve satisfactory reduction, fixation, and union. The

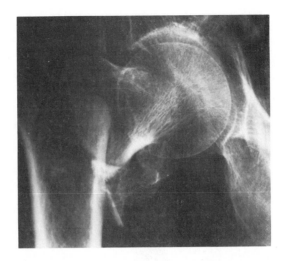

Fig. 21. Unstable intertrochanteric fracture. AP view of the hip showing the four-part fracture of the intertrochanteric region with comminution of the medial femoral cortex.

most commonly unappreciated components on the initial films are the size and degree of separation of the lesser trochanteric fragment, which represents a significant buttressing force on the posteromedial aspect of the femur.

Although the vast majority of extracapsular fractures will heal spontaneously, with a low incidence of avascular necrosis, surgery is recom-

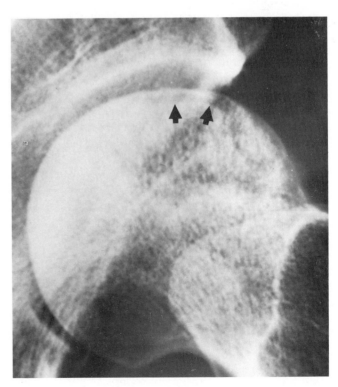

Fig. 22. Early aseptic necrosis. A fine radiolucent area (arrows) in the subchondral area of the femoral head indicates ischemic resorption.

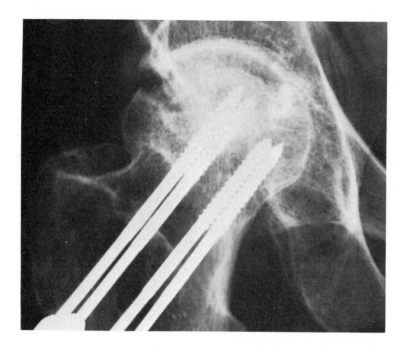

Fig. 23. Avascular necrosis, late stage. This AP view shows increased density of the femoral head and collapse of the articular surface.

mended in most cases to afford early patient mobilization. The unstable fracture is a serious problem with a much higher morbidity and mortality than the stable fracture. Surgery is difficult, and an osteotomy may be necessary with valgus repair to afford better stability.[12,63]

Isolated avulsion fractures of the greater or lesser trochanter are more frequent in children and in the young athletic adult. Operative treatment depends on the amount of displacement.

Complications

The most frequent complications of fractures of the proximal femur are aseptic necrosis of the femoral head, nonunion, degenerative arthritis, and infection. Aseptic necrosis is prevalent in intracapsular fractures but is rarely seen with those occurring outside the capsule. In nonstable intracapsular fractures the incidence of late aseptic necrosis rises from 25% with early treatment to 40% with 48-hr delay of therapy.[42] The earliest roentgen change may be a radiolucent crescent paralleling the articular margin of the femoral head (Fig. 22), indicating subchondral bone resorption. Areas of varying density may appear in the femoral head with preservation of the joint space. Ultimately there is collapse of the femoral head (Fig. 23), with severe degenerative arthritis. Necrosis and collapse involving the fracture surface may lead to failure of union, whereas collapse at the articular surface leads to degenerative arthritis.[1]

The incidence of avascular necrosis is higher histologically than radiographically.[30,55,67] Recently isotopic studies using ^{99m}Tc-diphosphonate and fluoride 18 have suggested that preoperative evaluation of the integrity of the blood supply of the femoral head following acute fracture may be possible.[10,11,78]

Nonunion is practically nonexistent in extracapsular fractures. The vast majority of examples of nonunion occur in intracapsular fractures and are associated with avascular necrosis of the femoral head.[60] Degenerative arthritis may result from mechanical damage to the articular cartilage at the time of injury or may be a consequence of poor vascular supply to the femoral head.

ACKNOWLEDGMENTS

Special thanks to Mrs. Marie McMurrey for her assistance in completing this paper and to Mrs. Kathryn Sisson for producing Fig. 11. Figures 1, 2, 5, 6, 7, 9, and 10 were reprinted with permission from the *Journal of Bone and Joint Surgery.*[14,37]

REFERENCES

1. Adams JC: Outline of Fractures, Including Joint Injuries (ed 6). Baltimore, Williams & Wilkins, 1972

2. Athanasoulis CA, Duffield R, Shapiro JH: Angiography to assess pelvic vascular injury. N Engl J Med 284:1329, 1971

3. Barnes R, Brown JT, Garden RS, et al: Subcapital fractures of the femur: A prospective review. J Bone Joint Surg [Br] 58:2–24, 1976

4. Barnes ST, Hinds RB: Pseudotumor of the ischium: A late manifestation of avulsion of the ischial epiphysis. J Bone Joint Surg [Am] 54:645–647, 1962

5. Ben-Menachem Y, Duke JH, Harberg BL, et al: Preoperative angiography in vascular trauma: Report of four unusual cases. J Trauma 15:209–216, 1975

6. Carey LS, Grace DM: The brisk bleed: Control by arterial catheterization and gelfoam plug. J Can Assoc Radiol 25:113–115, 1974

7. Cass AS: Bladder trauma in the multiple injured patient. J Urol 115:667–669, 1976

8. Clark SS, Prudencio RF: Lower urinary tract injuries associated with pelvic fractures. Diagnosis and management. Surg Clin North Am 52:183–201, 1972

9. Conolly WB, Hedberg EA: Observations on fractures of the pelvis. J Trauma 9:104–111, 1969

10. D'Ambrosia RD, Riggins RS, Stadalnik RC, et al: Experience with ^{99m}Tc diphosphonate in studying vascularity of the femoral head. Surg Forum 26:521–523, 1975

11. D'Ambrosia RD, Riggins RS, DeNardo SJ, et al: Fluoride-18 scintigraphy in avascular necrotic disorders of bone. Clin Orthop 107:146–155, 1975

12. Dimon JH, Hughston JC: Unstable intertrochanteric fractures of the hip. J Bone Joint Surg [Am] 49:440–450, 1967

13. Dommisse GF: Diametric fractures of the pelvis. J Bone Joint Surg [Br] 42:432–443, 1960

14. Dunn AW, Morris HD: Fractures and dislocations of the pelvis. J Bone Joint Surg [Am] 50:1639–1648, 1968

15. Duverney JG: Traite des Maladies de Os, vol. 1. Paris, De Bure l'Aîné, 1751

16. Ellis R, Green AG: Ischial apophyseolysis. Radiology 87:646–648, 1966

17. Epstein HC: Posterior fracture-dislocations of the hip: Long term follow-up. J Bone Joint Surg [Am] 56:1103–1127, 1974

18. Epstein HC: Traumatic dislocations of the hip. Clin Orthop 92:116–142, 1973

19. Fleming WH, Bowen JC 3rd: Control of hemorrhage in pelvic crush injuries. J Trauma 13:567–570, 1973

20. Furey WW: Fractures of the pelvis with special reference to associated fractures of the sacrum. Am J Roentgenol 47:89–96, 1942

21. Garden RS: Low-angle fixation in fractures of the femoral neck. J Bone Joint Surg [Br] 43:647–663, 1961

22. Garden RS: Reduction and fixation of subcapital fractures of the femur. Orthop Clin North Am 5:683–712, 1974

23. Garden RS: Stability and union in subcapital fractures of the femur. J Bone Joint Surg [Br] 46:630–647, 1964

24. Gerlock AJ: Hemorrhage following pelvic fracture controlled by embolization. Case report. J Trauma 15:740–742, 1975

25. Gilchrist MR, Peterson DH: Pelvic fracture and associated soft tissue trauma. Radiology 88:278–280, 1967

26. Griffiths WE, Swanson SA, Freeman MAR: Experimental fatigue fracture of the human cadaveric femoral neck. J Bone Joint Surg [Br] 53:136–143, 1971

27. Gyepes M, Mellins HZ, Katz I: The low incidence of fracture of the hip in the Negro. Practitioner 193:593–604, 1964

28. Hamsa WR: Epiphyseal injuries about the hip joint. Clin Orthop 10:119–124, 1957

29. Hauser CW, Perry JF Jr: Control of massive hemorrhage from pelvic fractures by hypogastric artery ligation. Surg Gynecol Obstet 121:313–315, 1965

30. Herndon JH, Aufranc OE: Avascular necrosis of the femora in the adult: A review of its incidence in a variety of conditions. Clin Orthop 86:43–62, 1972

31. Hewitt RL, Smith AD, Drapanas T: Acute traumatic arteriovenous fistulas. J Trauma 13:901–906, 1973

32. Holdsworth FW: Dislocation and fracture-dislocations of the pelvis. J Bone Joint Surg [Br] 30:461–466, 1948

33. Holm CL: Treatment of pelvic fractures and dislocations. Skeletal traction and the dual pelvic traction sling. Clin Orthop 97:97–107, 1973

34. Howard FM, Meany RP: Stress fracture of the pelvis during pregnancy. J Bone Joint Surg [Am] 43:538–540, 1961

35. Hunter GA: Posterior dislocations and fracture-dislocation of the hip. A review of fifty-seven patients. J Bone Joint Surg [Br] 51:38–44, 1969

36. Jeffery CC: Spontaneous fractures of the femoral neck. J Bone Joint Surg [Br] 44:543–549, 1962

37. Judet R, Judet J, Letournel E: Fractures of the acetabulum: Classification and surgical approaches for open reduction. J Bone Joint Surg [Am] 46:1615–1646, 1964

38. Linton P: On the different types of intracapsular fractures of the femoral neck. Acta Chir Scand [Suppl 90] 86:7–122, 1944

39. Malgaigne JF: Treatise on Fractures. Philadelphia, JB Lippincott, 1959

40. Margolies MN, Ring EJ, Waltman AC, et al: Arteriography in the management of hemorrhage from pelvic fractures. N Engl J Med 287:317–321, 1972

41. Mason ML: Intracapsular fractures of the neck of the femur. A review of 100 cases treated by internal fixation. Br J Surg 40:482–486, 1953

42. Massie WK: Treatment of femoral neck fracture emphasizing long term follow-up observations on aseptic necrosis. Clin Orthop 92:16–62, 1973

43. McElvenny RT: Roentgenographic interpretation of what constitutes adequate reduction of femoral neck fractures. Surg Gynecol Obstet 80:97–106, 1945

44. Medelman JP: Fractures of the sacrum: Their incidence in fracture of the pelvis. Am J Roentgenol 42:100–103, 1939

45. Motamed HA: Fractures of the acetabulum: Analysis of 59 cases. Int Surg 59:20–24, 1974

46. Motsay GJ, Alho A, Butler B, et al: Iliac vein trauma with pelvic fracture. Postgrad Med 51:133–136, 1972

47. Mounts RJ, Schloss CD: Injuries to the bony pelvis and hip. Radiol Clin North Am 4:307–322, 1966

48. Muecke EC, Currarino G: Congenital widening of the pubic symphysis. Associated clinical disorders and roentgen

anatomy of affected bony pelves. Am J. Roentgenol 103:179–185, 1968

49. Newton-John HF, Morgan DB: The loss of bone with age, osteoporosis, and fractures. Clin Orthop 71:229–252, 1970

50. Nilsson BE, Hagberg L: Proceedings: Prediction of femoral neck fracture from a pelvic x-ray. Am J Roentgenol 126:1299–1300, 1976

51. Northrop CH, Eto RT, Loop JW: Vertical fracture of the sacral ala. Significance of non-continuity of the anterior superior sacral foraminal line. Am J Roentgenol 124:102–106, 1975

52. Patterson FP, Morton KS: The cause of death in fractures of the pelvis, with a note on treatment by ligation of the hypogastric (internal iliac) artery. J Trauma 13:849–856, 1973

53. Peltier LF: Complications associated with fractures of the pelvis. J Bone Joint Surg [Am] 47:1060–1069, 1965

54. Pennal GF, Sutherland G: Fractures of the pelvis (motion picture available from any film library of The American Academy of Orthopedic Surgeons). 1961

55. Phemister DB: Fractures of neck of femur, dislocations of hip, and obscure vascular disturbances producing aseptic necrosis of head of femur. Surg Gynecol Obstet 59:415–440, 1934

56. Rankin LM: Fractures of the pelvis. A review of 449 cases. Ann Surg 106:266–277, 1937

57. Reynolds BM, Balsano NA: Venography in pelvic fractures. A clinical evaluation. Ann Surg 173:104–106, 1971

58. Reynolds BM, Balsano NA, Reynolds FS: Pelvic fractures. J Trauma 13:1011–1014, 1973

59. Ring EJ, Waltman AC, Athanasoulis C, et al: Angiography in pelvic trauma. Surg Gynecol Obstet 139:375–380, 1974

60. Rockwood CA Jr, Green DP: Fractures, vol. 2. Philadelphia, JB Lippincott, 1975

61. Rogers LF, Novy SB, Harris NF: Occult central fractures of the acetabulum. Am J Roentgenol 124:96–101, 1975

62. Rowe CR, Lowell JD: Prognosis of fractures of the acetabulum. J Bone Joint Surg [Am] 43:30–59, 1961

63. Sarmiento A, Williams, EM: The unstable intertrochanteric fracture: Treatment with a valgus osteotomy

and I-beam nail-plate. A preliminary report of one hundred cases. J Bone Joint Surg [Am] 52:1309–1318, 1970

64. Scheck M: Intracapsular fracture of the femoral neck. Comminution of the posterior neck cortex as a cause of unstable fixation. J Bone Joint Surg [Am] 41:1187–1200, 1959

65. Schneider R, Kay J, Ghelman B: Adductor avulsive injuries near the symphisis pubis. Radiology 120:567–569, 1976

66. Selakovich W, Love L: Stress fractures of the pubic ramus. J Bone Joint Surg [Am] 36:573–576, 1954

67. Sevitt S: Avascular necrosis and revascularisation of the femoral head after intracapsular fractures. A combined arteriographic and histological necropsy study. J Bone Joint Surg [Br] 46:270–296, 1964

68. Smith GR, Loop JW: Radiologic classification of posterior dislocations of the hip: Refinements and pitfalls. Radiology 119:569–574, 1976

69. Smith K, Ben-Menachem Y, Duke JH, et al: The superior gluteal: An artery at risk in blunt pelvic trauma. J Trauma 16:273–279, 1976

70. Stayton CA Jr: Ischial epiphysiolysis. Am J Roentgenol 76:1161–1162, 1956

71. Treasure R: Spontaneous fractures of the pelvis in middle-aged women. J Bone Joint Surg [Br] 45:223, 1963

72. Tronzo RG: Special considerations in management (symposium on fractures of the hip, pt I). Orthop Clin North Am 5:571–583, 1974

73. Trunkey DD, Chapman MW, Lim RC, et al: Management of pelvic fractures in blunt trauma injury. J Trauma 14:912–923, 1974

74. Vix VA, Ryu CY: The adult symphysis pubis: Normal and abnormal. Am J Roentgenol 112:517–525, 1971

75. Vose GP, Lockwood RM: Femoral neck fracturing—Its relationship to radiographic bone density. J Gerontol 20:300–305, 1965

76. Wakeley CPG: Fractures of the pelvis: An analysis of 100 cases. Br J Surg 17:22–29, 1930

77. Watson-Jones R: Fractures and Joint Injuries, vol. 2 (ed 4). Baltimore, Williams & Wilkins, 1955

78. Webber MM, Wagner J, Cragin MD, et al: Femoral head blood supply demonstrated by radiotracers. Proceedings of 21st Annual Meeting, Society of Nuclear Medicine. J Nucl Med 15:543, 1974 (abstract)

Knee

Kakarla Subbarao and Harold G. Jacobson

THE KNEE JOINT has evolved into a highly specialized structure in the human, surpassing that of all lower animals in its complexity. The cause lies in the excessive functional demands made on the human knee as a result of man's erect posture. Weight-bearing, walking, running, and the ability to extend the knee completely are physiologic functions that subject the human knee to considerably more stress than in four-legged mammals.

The knee, the largest joint in the body, is in a vulnerable position for direct trauma and unusual torsional and bending stresses. The security of the knee depends mostly on the powerful ligaments that bind the osseous components together, as well as on the muscles that surround it. Increasing participation in various sports activities has subjected more and more individuals to greater stress and severe injury of the knees than ever before.

Detailed knowledge of the radiologic anatomy of the knee is important for complete understanding of the mechanisms of the injuries involving specific bony parts. Injuries to menisci, ligaments, tendons, and muscles, with or without osteochondral fractures, are not uncommon. The medial and lateral menisci, the medial and lateral collateral ligaments, the cruciate ligaments, the attachment sites of important muscles, eg, the quadriceps and the biceps femoris, constitute critical structures in radiologic anatomy. Figure 1 illustrates the important areas of the knee to be considered radiologically.

From a radiologic point of view, a traumatized knee demands the utmost care in demonstrating the injury with least discomfort and inconvenience to the patient. PA or AP and lateral views of the knee constitute a basic minimum in the radiologic examination. Additional projections, such as oblique, tunnel, and skyline views, horizontal beam films, stress films, and tomograms, are often necessary alone or in combination.

On occasion, a follow-up film after an interval of 10 to 14 days may be valuable in establishing the diagnosis by demonstrating periosteal reaction or callus and revealing resorption of bone around the margins of fracture fragments. Isotopic scanning studies using technetium pyrophosphate may also be helpful, particularly in confirming the presence of stress fracture or other subtle fractures. On occasion, arthrography may clearly demonstrate a depressed fracture of the tibial plateau, loose fragments of bone, and cartilage and meniscal injuries.[1]

FRACTURES OF DISTAL FEMORAL CONDYLES

Types

Fractures of the distal femoral condyles are uncommon. Three major types exist (Fig. 2):[15]

I. Sagittal, with part or all of the condyle split from the femoral shaft.

II. Coronal, with the posterior condyle displaced.

III. A combination of sagittal and coronal fractures.

Overlap of these three types is common.

Mechanism

Hyperabduction or adduction forces with axial loading from weight-bearing may avulse an entire femoral condyle or a portion of it.

Radiologic Features

Tangential or oblique views of the knee may be necessary to accurately demonstrate the extent of the fracture and the degree of displacement of the fractured condyle so as to ensure proper treatment. If the films are adequate, there should be no difficulty in establishing the diagnosis.

Kakarla Subbarao, M.D.: *Associate Professor of Radiology;* Harold G. Jacobson, M.D.: *Professor and Chairman, Department of Radiology; Albert Einstein College of Medicine, Montefiore Hospital and Medical Center, Bronx, N.Y.*

Reprint requests should be addressed to Kakarla Subbarao, M.D., Department of Radiology, Albert Einstein College of Medicine, Montefiore Hospital and Medical Center, 111 East 210th Street, Bronx, N.Y. 10467.

© *1978 by Grune & Stratton, Inc.*

0037-198X/78/1302-0007$0100/0

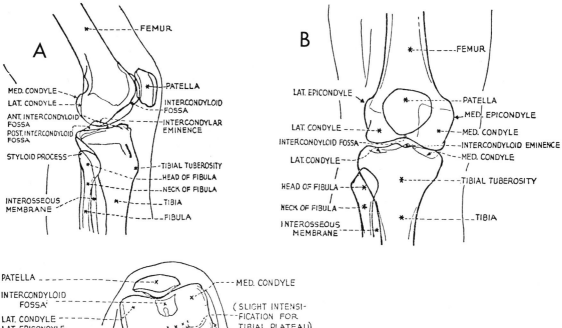

A

FEMUR
MED. CONDYLE
LAT. CONDYLE
ANT. INTERCONDYLOID FOSSA
POST. INTERCONDYLOID FOSSA
STYLOID PROCESS
INTEROSSEOUS MEMBRANE
PATELLA
INTERCONDYLOID FOSSA
INTERCONDYLAR EMINENCE
TIBIAL TUBEROSITY
HEAD OF FIBULA
NECK OF FIBULA
TIBIA
FIBULA

B

FEMUR
LAT. EPICONDYLE
LAT. CONDYLE
INTERCONDYLOID FOSSA
LAT. CONDYLE
HEAD OF FIBULA
NECK OF FIBULA
INTEROSSEOUS MEMBRANE
PATELLA
MED. EPICONDYLE
MED. CONDYLE
INTERCONDYLOID EMINENCE
MED. CONDYLE
TIBIAL TUBEROSITY
TIBIA

C

PATELLA
INTERCONDYLOID FOSSA
LAT. CONDYLE
LAT. EPICONDYLE
STYLOID PROCESS
HEAD OF FIBULA
TIBIAL TUBEROSITY
NECK OF FIBULA
MED. CONDYLE
(SLIGHT INTENSIFICATION FOR TIBIAL PLATEAU)
MED. EPICONDYLE
BODY OF TIBIA
BODY OF FEMUR

Fig. 1. Diagrammatic anatomic sketches of the normal knee in the lateral, AP, and patellar views. (Reproduced by permission from Meschan I: An Atlas of Anatomy Basic to Radiology. Philadelphia, WB Saunders, 1975.)

Fig. 2. Diagrammatic sketches of the types of fracture of the distal femoral condyles. [Reproduced by permission from Rockwood CA Jr, Green DP (eds): Fractures. Philadelphia, JB Lippincott, 1975.]

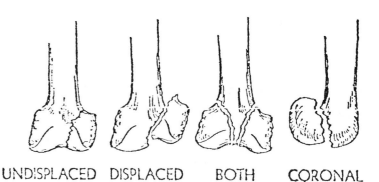

UNDISPLACED   DISPLACED   BOTH CONDYLES   CORONAL

FRACTURES OF TIBIAL CONDYLES

Types

Hohl's classification[5] (Fig. 3) is probably the most pragmatic, although it is designed primarily for therapeutic purposes:

I. Undisplaced
II. Local compression
III. Split compression
IV. Total condylar depression
V. Split fracture
VI. Comminuted

Mechanism

The mechanism of injury generally relates to a forcible thrust of the femoral condyle against the tibial plateau. Depending on the force of impact, the tibial condyle may show compression, comminution, or splitting.

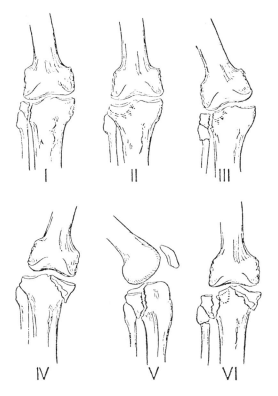

Fig. 3. Diagrammatic sketch of the six types of fracture of the tibial condyles: I. Undisplaced. II. Local compression. III. Split compression. IV. Total condylar depression. V. Split fracture. VI. Comminuted. From Hohl M.[5]

Radiologic Features

An undisplaced fracture shows less than 4 mm of compression or condylar space widening.[12] An important issue is the high incidence of ligamentous avulsions along the tibial surfaces or the head of the fibula. Stress films often are helpful in demonstrating these avulsions. As an example, a fracture of the lateral tibial condyle (Segond fracture) with an avulsion at the bony insertion of the tensor fascia lata (iliotibial band) is optimally demonstrated by varus (adduction) stress on the knee.

Compression fractures are divided into two distinct subtypes. Local compression fracture is a depressed condylar fracture shaped like the femoral condyle that produced it. The second subtype is the compressed fracture of the lateral tibial plateau, also referred to as "bumper" or "fender" fracture (Fig. 4).

The split compression fracture is characterized by compression in the middle of the articular surface of the tibia, as well as a peripheral split fragment with intact articular cartilage and cortex.

The total condylar depression fracture is observed frequently to involve the medial condyle, without significant articular surface damage. The fracture line enters the area of the intercondylar eminence.

The split fracture, which is uncommon, differs from the split compression fracture in that there is no associated articular surface compression. These fractures of the articular margin usually shear off the anterior or posterior aspect of the medial tibial condyle. The radiologic features are characteristic.

A comminuted fracture has an ominous appearance because of the marked distortion of the upper tibial articular surfaces. However, many comminuted fractures realign and remodel satisfactorily after the application of skeletal traction. They involve both tibial

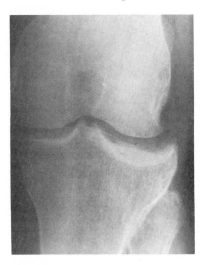

Fig. 4. Compressed fracture of the lateral tibial condyle (plateau) is shown.

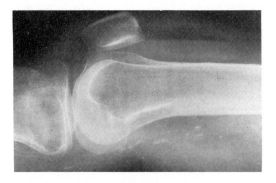

Fig. 5. Horizontal beam film demonstrating a fat–fluid level in a patient with compression fractures of both tibial condyles.

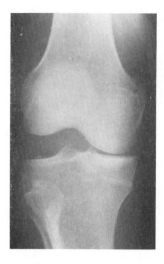

Fig. 6. Varus (adduction) stress film shows marked widening of the lateral knee joint cartilage indicating rupture of the lateral ligament. A chip fracture of the lateral tibial condyle is present.

condyles, producing a wide variety of configurations, accompanied by depression of each condyle with damage of the articular surfaces.

Routine AP and lateral views of the knee are adequate to demonstrate the presence of most tibial condylar fractures. However, on occasion a fracture can only be identified on oblique projections or by laminagraphy.

The demonstration of a fat–fluid level with a horizontal beam film virtually mandates obtaining additional views of the knee if a fracture is not demonstrated on the standard projections (Fig. 5). Thus, valgus and varus stress films are recommended with trauma known to produce a high incidence of associated ligamentous injuries, eg, compression and undisplaced fractures (Fig. 6). Anesthesia, regional or general, is recommended when stress films are considered essential. Stress is applied to the knee in full extension and in approximately 15 degrees flexion. A special 10-degree caudal AP view of the knee should be used when an accurate determination of the amount of articular depression is needed to determine the proper method of treatment.[15] Arthrography may also be helpful in delineating traumatic capsular and ligamentous defects.

FRACTURES OF TIBIAL SPINE

Fracture of either of the tibial spines, or more commonly of the entire intercondylar eminence, indicates structural damage of the anterior cruciate ligament.[8,11] Interference with full ex-

tension of the knee may be caused by displacement of bone fragments, requiring surgical correction. In fact, most of the loose bodies encountered in the knee joint either originate from the tibial spines or represent osteochondral fractures from the articulating margins of the femoral or tibial condyles or patella.

Types

Fractures of the intercondylar eminence are classified by the degree of displacement of the fractured fragment,[15] as illustrated in Fig. 7:

I. The fragment is tilted up only on the anterior margin.

II. The anterior portion is lifted up completely from its bed, with only some posterior apposition.

IIIA. The intercondylar fragment is not in contact with the tibia.

IIIB. The intercondylar fragment is rotated.

Mechanism

Most of the injuries are due to violent twisting of the knee or to an abduction-adduction injury. In some instances, direct contact with the adjacent femoral condyle is responsible. In addition to the tear of the anterior cruciate ligament and tibial spine fracture, other osseous structures may be fractured.[8]

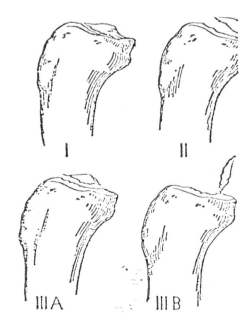

Fig. 7. Schematic classification of fractures of the intercondylar eminence. From Meyers, MH and McKeever FMJ.[11]

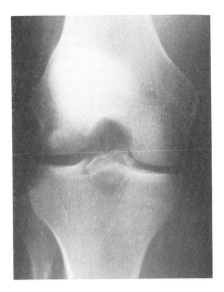

Fig. 8. Fracture of the entire intercondylar eminence shown on tunnel view. The fracture implies a serious injury to the anterior cruciate ligament.

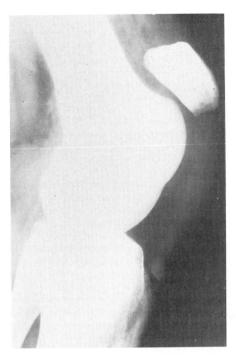

Fig. 9. Avulsion fracture of the anterior tibial tubercle with upward dislocation of the patella, caused by rupture of the infrapatellar tendon and contracture of the quadriceps tendon.

Radiologic Features

Although routine films of the knee generally demonstrate the fracture, a tunnel view is helpful in outlining the position of the fragment (Fig. 8). Other areas of ligamentous attachment must be scrutinized for additional avulsion fractures.

FRACTURE OF TIBIAL TUBEROSITY

Fracture of the tibial tuberosity is not an uncommon isolated injury, but it is more often observed in association with comminuted or subcondylar fracture of the proximal end of the tibia. Since the tibial tuberosity provides insertion for the quadriceps mechanism through the patellar tendon, the correct diagnosis is essential for proper treatment.

Mechanism

Tibial tuberosity fracture often takes place during athletic activities in which indirect violence occurs with the knee flexed and the quadriceps tendon firmly resisting further flexion.[4] The range of maximum tensile stress of the tendon may be considerably greater than the tensile stress in the resting state in many sports situations.

Radiologic Features

In isolated fracture of the tibial tuberosity, the tuberosity necessarily is avulsed and dis-

placed proximally. With associated rupture of the infrapatellar tendon, the patella is dislocated upward by the contracture of the quadriceps tendon (Fig. 9). Hemarthrosis is evident in routine views. The triangular fat pad posterior to the patellar tendon is obliterated.

FRACTURES OF PATELLA

Fractures of the patella are common, occurring at any age[3] (Fig. 10).

Types[15]

I. Transverse or oblique
   A. Fragments of equal size
   B. Small upper fragment
   C. Smaller lower fragment
II. Comminuted or stellate
III. Polar
IV. Vertical
V. Marginal
VI. Osteochondral

Mechanism

Patellar fractures are produced by either direct or indirect forces. A fracture caused by indirect force is associated with violent pull of

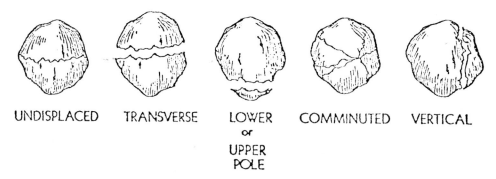

UNDISPLACED   TRANSVERSE   LOWER   COMMINUTED   VERTICAL
                                 or
                             UPPER
                             POLE

Fig. 10.   Schematic sketch of the types of patellar fracture.

the musculotendinous insertion, and typically occurs during the act of stumbling down stairs or an incline. These fractures are usually transverse, often with some degree of comminution. The degree of separation of the proximal and distal poles of the patella depends on the extent of tear of the quadriceps expansion.

A fracture due to direct force is brought about by the patella striking a solid object, such as a dashboard, or being traumatized in a fall on a hard surface. These fractures are incomplete or undisplaced, stellate or comminuted.

Combined direct and indirect injuries occur and are characterized by considerable separation of fragments, indicative of tear of the medial and lateral quadriceps expansion.

Radiologic Features

Besides the standard projections of the knee, a "skyline" view of the patella is essential. This film helps to identify small osteochondral fractures, marginal chip fractures, and vertical fractures that can be easily overlooked in the AP and lateral views. However, the skyline view

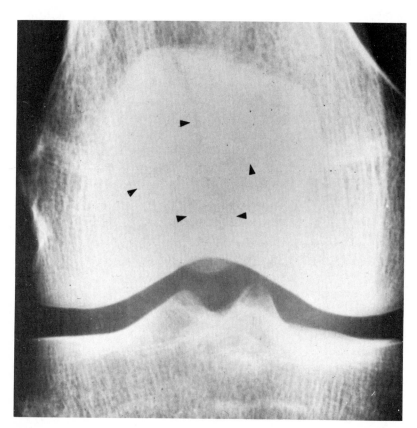

Fig. 11.   Stellate fracture of the patella shown on an AP film of the knee.

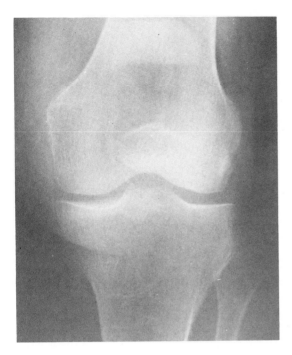

Fig. 12. Complete transverse fracture of the patella, with wide separation of fragments shown on an AP view.

may be difficult to obtain in a traumatized patient with considerable pain and limitation of motion. In such patients, a well-penetrated AP film may afford sufficient detail of the patella through the superimposed distal femur to diagnose a stellate or transverse fracture (Figs. 11 and 12). The lateral view is important, since it profiles the patella and outlines the continuity of its articular surface, permitting assessment of patellar displacement.

The marginal and osteochondral ("flake") fractures of the patella are often associated with recurrent dislocation of the patella (Fig. 13). This association is important, particularly with osteochondral fractures involving the inferior medial borders of the patella.

The differential diagnosis of patellar fractures principally involves congenital anomalies of the patella, especially a bipartite or tripartite patella. These accessory ossicles have well-defined cortical margins and are invariably located on the superior lateral border of the patella. They are often bilateral, so that a comparison view of the uninjured knee is generally helpful.

FRACTURES OF PROXIMAL END OF FIBULA

Fracture of the proximal end of the fibula is usually relatively unimportant. However, associated complications, such as injury to the peroneal nerve and anterior tibial artery, should be sought. Avulsion fracture of the styloid process of the fibula is particularly important, since it is associated with rupture of the biceps tendon (Fig. 14). An associated tibiofibular ligamentous injury will produce lateral instability.

Mechanism

Three major types of injury produce fracture of the proximal end of the fibula:[15]

A. Direct blow
B. Twisting injury at the ankle
C. Varus (adduction) stress to the knee

A fracture of the fibular head resulting from a direct blow is usually comminuted but not displaced. A fracture below the head of the fibula should always create suspicion of an associated fracture at the ankle joint, usually due to an external rotation injury. This combination is often encountered in parachutists. Fibular fractures are relatively silent, producing few symptoms.

Fig. 13. Skyline view of the patella, showing marginal fractures of both its lateral and medial surfaces, with lateral subluxation of the patella.

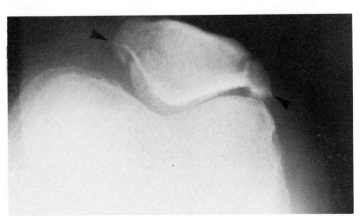

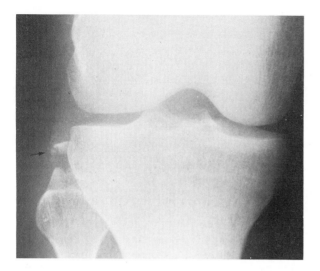

Fig. 14. Avulsion fracture of the styloid process of the fibula, which is associated with rupture of the biceps tendon.

Fracture of the fibular head or styloid process produced by varus stress is an important injury. Depending on the severity of the trauma, the lateral collateral ligament may be ruptured or the common peroneal nerve may be stretched or torn. *Lateral compartment syndrome of the knee* and *ligamentous peroneal nerve syndrome* are names that have been coined to describe the association of an adduction stress to the knee, rupture of the capsular and ligamentous structures, and a peroneal nerve injury. When produced by a severe valgus stress, fracture of the head of the fibula may be associated with a lateral tibial condylar fracture.

Radiologic Features

Apart from the standard routine projections of the knee, stress films are essential to demonstrate the associated ligamentous injury (Fig. 6). The diagnosis of fracture of the fibular head is generally not difficult. However, a chip

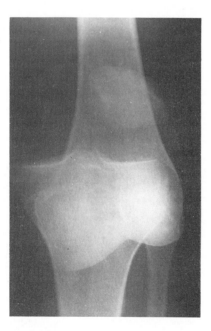

Fig. 15. Anterior dislocation at the femorotibial joint, with the tibia and fibula overlapping the femoral condyles. AP view of the knee.

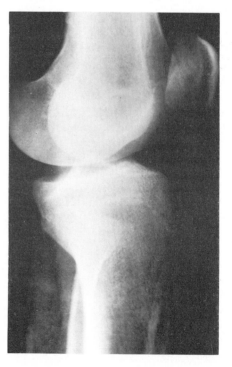

Fig. 16. Anterior dislocation of the head of the fibula. The head of the fibula overlaps the tibia in the lateral view of the knee.

fracture of the styloid process of the fibula associated with rupture of the biceps tendon is not always easy to identify. The small bone fragment may be mistaken for tendinous or ligamentous calcification. On occasion, a chip fracture may be obscured by the lateral condyle of the tibia, in which instance oblique views are of help in delineating the fragment.

DISLOCATIONS AROUND KNEE

Dislocations around the knee occur at three joints, the patellofemoral joint, the femorotibial joint, and the proximal tibiofibular joint. Dislocation at the patellofemoral joint is either congenital or acquired; the latter is predominantly traumatic. The acute traumatic type comprises lateral, vertical, interarticular, and intercondylar dislocations. Recurrent and habitual subluxations occur with an underlying congenital deficiency, either of the patella or of the lateral condyle, but trauma precipitates the dislocation. The importance of radiologic

study is to detect osteochondral fracture associated with the dislocated patella (Fig. 13).

Dislocations at the femorotibial joint are either anterior or posterior (Fig. 15). These dislocations are also described as open, closed, or isolated dislocation, or fracture dislocation. A major violence in an automobile accident or a fall from a height is the usual cause. In both anterior and posterior dislocations, one or both cruciate ligaments are torn. In some instances, injury to the popliteal artery or peroneal nerve may occur.

Dislocations at the proximal tibiofibular joint are classified as anterior, posterior, or superior. In the anterior dislocation (Fig. 16) the head of the fibula is also dislocated slightly laterally, whereas in the posterior dislocation the head of the fibula is dislocated slightly medially. In all dislocations, the ankle should always be included in the radiographic examination to rule out associated injuries. In superior dislocation of the head of the fibula, upward displacement of the lateral malleolus is always present.

REFERENCES

1. Anderson PW, Harley JD, Maslin, PU: Arthrographic evaluation of problems with united tibial plateau fractures. Radiology 119:75–78, 1976

2. Cave EF, Nicholson JT, West FE, MacAusland WR, Jr. et al: Symposium on fractures about the knee. American Academy of Orthopedic Surgeons Instructional Course Lecture, 18:73–91, 1961

3. Griswold AS: Fractures of the patella. Clin Orthoped 4:44–56, 1954

4. Hand WL, Hand CR, Dunn AW: Avulsion fractures of the tibial tubercle. J Bone Joint Surg 53A:1579–1583, 1971

5. Hohl M: Tibial condylar fractures. J Bone Joint Surg 49A:1455–1467, 1967

6. Jacobson HG: American College of Radiology Seminars on Trauma. Presented in Atlanta, Feb. 1977

7. Kennedy JC, Grainger RW, McGraw RW: Osteochondral fractures of the femoral condyles. J Bone and Joint Surgery 48B:436–440, 1966

8. Liljedahl SO, Lindvall N, Wetterfors J: Roentgen diagnosis of rupture of anterior cruciate ligament. Acta Radiol. (Stockholm) 4:225–239, 1966

9. Lucht U, Pilgaard S: Fractures of the tibial condyles. Acta Orthop. Scand. 42:366–376, 1971

10. Martin AF: The pathomechanics of the knee joint. The medial collateral ligament and lateral tibial plateau fractures. J Bone and Joint Surg. 42A:13–22, 1960

11. Meyers MH, McKeever FM: Fracture of the intercondylar eminence of the tibia. J Bone Joint Surg 52A:1677–1684, 1970

12. Moore TM, Harvey JP Jr.: Roentgenographic measurement of tibial-plateau depression due to fracture. J Bone Joint Surg 56A:155–160, 1974

13. Porter BB: Crush fractures of the lateral tibial table. Factors influencing the prognosis. J Bone Joint Surg 52B:676–687, 1970

14. Rasmussen PS: Tibial condylar fractures. Impairmen of knee joint stability as an indication for surgical treatment J Bone and Joint Surgery 53A:1331–1350, 1973

15. Rockwood CA, Jr., Green DP: Fractures. Vol. 2, Philadelphia, Lippincott, 1975

16. Shelton ME, Neer CS II, Grantham SA: Occult-knee ligament rupture associated with fractures. J Trauma 11:853–856, 1971

17. Wilppula AE, Bakalim G: Ligamentous tear concomitant with tibial condular fracture. Acta Orthop. Scand. 43:292–300, 1972

Ankle

Jack Edeiken and Jerome M. Cotler

THE ANKLE bears more weight per unit area than any other joint. If there is contour disruption or instability, degenerative changes will occur. Fracture and dislocation reduction must be almost anatomically perfect, and ligamentous rupture must be adequately immobilized or surgically repaired. Ligaments may be injured in the absence of fracture, and they are as important in maintaining the ankle mortise as the skeletal structures. The radiologist usually concerns himself with the evaluation of the roentgenograms for fracture and dislocation, and the mechanism of injury and the ligamentous damage are largely ignored. Ligamentous damage unassociated with fracture is especially dangerous because it may go unrecognized and untreated.

The type of fracture (oblique or transverse) will usually indicate the mechanism and the potential ligamentous damage. In the absence of fracture or obvious dislocation, considerable soft-tissue swelling is an indication for stress studies to evaluate the ligamentous damage.

ANATOMY

The structures of the ankle may be compared to the mortise and tenon junction of a piece of furniture. The mortise is formed by the distal end of the tibia and the two malleoli. The distal tibial articular surface is called the plafond (ceiling) and is continuous with the medial malleolus where it courses inferomedially. The junction of the plafond and the medial malleolus is important, since fractures through or above it are usually unstable (Fig. 1). The tenon is the superior part of the talus. The articular surfaces of the tibia and talus narrow from anterior to posterior, which prevents posterior dislocation unless the mortise is disrupted (Fig. 2). The lateral malleolus (fibula) is in a plane about 1 cm distal and posterior to the medial malleolus. The talus articulates with the plafond superiorly and medially, and with the lateral malleolus.

The important ligaments of the ankle joint are the lateral collateral ligaments, the medial (deltoid) ligament, and the tibiofibular ligaments (or tibiofibular syndesmosis). Each ligament complex is composed of several bands. The lateral collateral ligaments consist of three

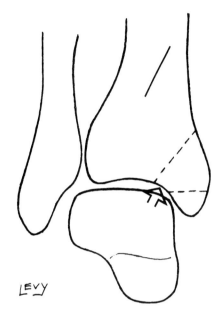

Fig. 1. Diagram of ankle joint. The junction of the plafond and the medial malleolus is important (arrow). Fractures at or above this junction are usually unstable; fractures below the junction are stable.

components: (1) the anterior talofibular ligament, which courses horizontally and anteriorly from the fibula to the talus; (2) the posterior talofibular ligament, which runs horizontally from the malleolus to the talus; (3) the calcaneofibular ligament, which courses inferiorly and posteriorly from the tip of the malleolus to the calcaneus between the two horizontal ligaments (Fig. 3). The stronger medial collateral (deltoid) ligament is composed of a thick triangular band consisting of two sets of fibers, superficial and deep. The superficial fibers run vertically from the tip of the malleolus and attach to the navicular, the sustentaculum tali of the calcaneus, and the talus (Fig. 4). The

Jack Edeiken, M.D.: *Department of Radiology;* Jerome M. Cotler, M.D.: *Department of Orthopedic Surgery; Thomas Jefferson University Hospital, Philadelphia, Pa.*

Reprint requests should be addressed to Jack Edeiken, M.D., Department of Radiology, Thomas Jefferson University Hospital, 11th and Walnut Streets, Philadelphia, Pa. 19107.

© *1978 by Grune & Stratton, Inc.*

0037-198X/78/1302-0008$0100/0

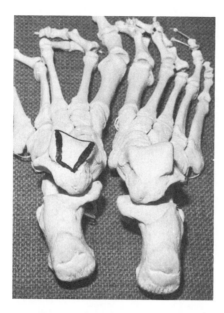

Fig. 2. Bilateral ankle joint specimens. The articular surface of the talus narrows posteriorly. This prevents posterior dislocation unless the mortise is disrupted. The superior articulating surface of the talus has been drawn on the left foot.

deep fibers run horizontally from the malleolus to the talus.

The distal tibia and fibula are bound by four ligaments: the anterior tibiofibular, the posterior tibiofibular, the inferior transverse, and the interosseous, which is the distal extension of

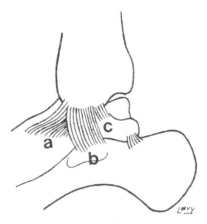

Fig. 4. The superficial fibers of the medial collateral (deltoid) ligament. (a) Band running from the malleolus to the navicular; (b) band from the malleolus to the sustentaculum tali; (c) band to the talus.

the interosseous membrane and is the strongest attachment of the tibia to the fibula (Fig. 5).

ROENTGEN EXAMINATION

AP and lateral views are the minimum requirements for examination of the ankle. With obvious fractures these may suffice, but oblique views may be necessary.

The AP view must be obtained with 5–15 degrees of adduction of the foot, or the distal tibia will obscure the lateral ankle joint. This is

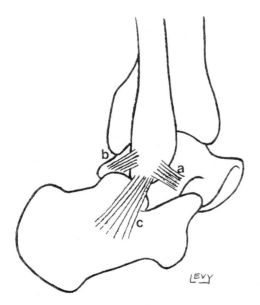

Fig. 3. The lateral collateral ligaments consist of three components: (a) the anterior talofibular, (b) the posterior talofibular, and (c) the calcaneofibular ligaments.

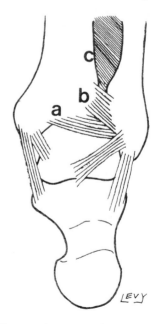

Fig. 5. The posterior aspect of the ankle and the posterior tibiofibular ligaments: (a) the inferior transverse ligament, (b) the interosseous ligament, and (c) the interosseous membrane.

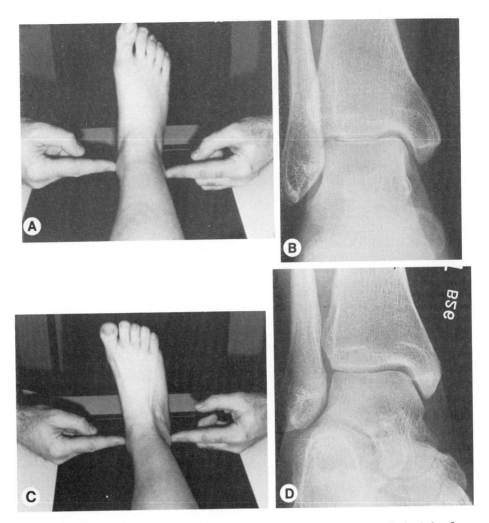

Fig. 6. The mortise view. (A) With the foot at a 90-degree angle to the table, the lateral malleolus is 1 to 2 cm posterior to the medial malleolus. (B) On the roentgenogram, the fibula obscures the lateral ankle joint. (C) With adduction of the foot (5–15 degrees) the malleoli are level. (D) On the roentgenogram, the lateral joint is opened. This is the mortise view.

called the mortise view (Fig. 6). The lateral malleolus lies 1 to 2 cm posterior to the medial malleolus, and adduction (internal rotation) rotates malleoli to the same horizontal plane, providing a satisfactory mortise view (Fig. 6D).

Stress films should be obtained when there is considerable soft-tissue swelling or pain in the absence of fractures. They are used to identify complete ligamentous tears. They are performed by adducting or abducting the heel. Local anesthesia may be necessary (Fig. 7).

The basic mechanisms of injury are inversion and eversion. It is recognized that other forces may complicate the basic mechanism; these include rotation, supination, pronation, and vertical compression.

INVERSION INJURIES

With forceful inversion of the foot, avulsion forces affect the lateral structures, and impactive forces (by the talar shift) stress the medial structures. Lateral injuries consist of one of the following: (1) sprain of the lateral collateral ligament, (2) avulsion of the lateral collateral ligament, (3) rupture of the lateral collateral ligament, or (4) transverse fracture of the lateral malleolus (Fig. 8). The only impacting injury to the medial structures is an oblique or spiral fracture of the medial malleolus (Fig. 9). Inversion injuries do not damage the tibiofibular or medial collateral ligaments.

With inversion, the first stress is placed on

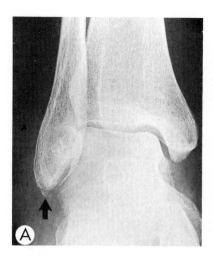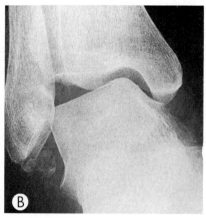

Fig. 7. Stress views. (A) Standard AP projection. A small chip fracture (arrow) is present at the distal end of the fibula. (B) Stress view in adduction reveals an abnormal tilt to the talus, indicating avulsion of the lateral collateral ligament. The fracture is better demonstrated.

the lateral part of the joint, and one of the four types of injury shown in Fig. 8 may occur. The talus then tends to dislocate and impact on the medial malleolus. If the impacting force is great enough, an oblique or spiral fracture of the medial malleolus occurs. In general, oblique or spiral fractures are due to impacting forces, and transverse fractures are due to avulsing forces. Thus the mechanism of injury may be deduced from the type of fracture (Fig. 10).

A medial malleolar fracture will not occur with a sprain of the lateral collateral ligament

and need not occur with the other three types of injury of the lateral joint structures.

Sprain of Lateral Collateral Ligament

Sprain of the lateral collateral ligament is a frequent injury. It is due to tearing of some of the ligament fibers, but the continuity of the ligament remains intact. The only roentgen finding with sprain is soft-tissue swelling, most marked distal to the lateral malleolus. Stress films will be normal. In obtaining stress films, it is important to compare both ankles, for as

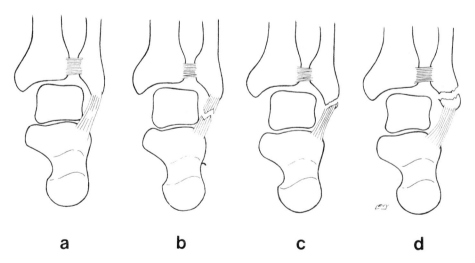

a   b   c   d

Fig. 8. Inversion injury. Avulsion stress on the lateral collateral ligament may cause (a) sprain of the lateral collateral ligament, (b) rupture of the body of the lateral collateral ligament, (c) avulsion of the lateral collateral ligament, or (d) transverse fracture of the lateral malleolus. The stresses of inversion injury do not affect the tibiofibular ligament or medial collateral ligament.

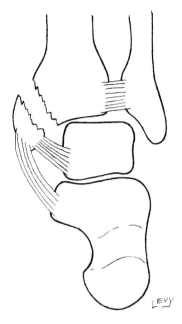

Fig. 9. The impacting force of an inversion injury may cause an oblique or spiral fracture of the medial malleolus.

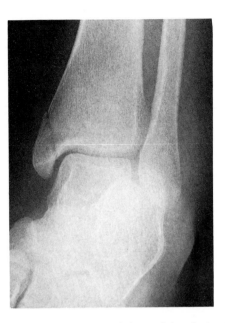

Fig. 11. Oblique fracture of the medial malleolus. This indicates an inversion injury. Since there is no fracture of the fibula, a rupture of the lateral collateral ligament must be present. Stress films are not necessary.

much as 15 degrees of angulation of the talus may occur normally.

Avulsion of Lateral Collateral Ligament

When the inversion force is great enough, the lateral collateral ligament may be avulsed from its attachment to the lateral malleolus. One or

more small chips of bone may be pulled from the tip of the malleolus (the so-called chip or sprain fracture). They indicate significant avulsion, and adequate immobilization is indicated. The roentgen features consist of severe soft-tissue swelling, most marked over the distal end of the fibula, and small chips of bone pulled from the lateral malleolus and sometimes the

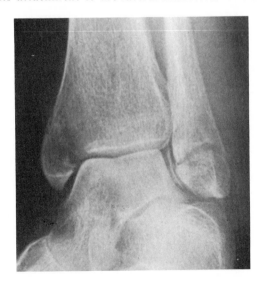

Fig. 10. An inversion injury of the ankle. There is an oblique fracture of the medial malleolus and a transverse fracture of the lateral malleolus. Oblique fractures indicate impaction, and transverse fractures indicate an avulsive force.

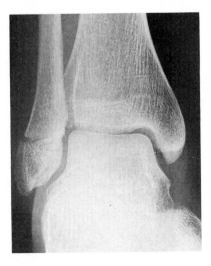

Fig. 12. Inversion injury. There is a transverse fracture of the lateral malleolus indicating avulsive forces. There is no lateral collateral ligament tear because the fracture has taken the brunt of the force.

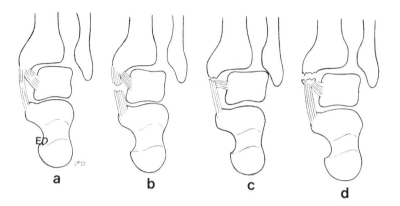

Fig. 13. Eversion injuries. Types of avulsive stress on the medial joint structures: (a) sprain of the deltoid ligament; (b) rupture of the deltoid ligament; (c) avulsion of the deltoid ligament; (d) transverse fracture of the medial malleolus.

talus (Fig. 7). Stress films are not necessary if a fresh fracture is identified.

Rupture of Lateral Collateral Ligament

In rupture of the lateral collateral ligament, the tear is away from the attachment to bone, and no fracture occurs. The roentgen features are the same as in sprain, with soft-tissue swelling most marked below the lateral malleolus. Stress films may be required to show the injury. They are unnecessary if clinical instability is apparent. If there is an associated oblique or spiral fracture of the medial malleolus, stress films are also unnecessary, for this indicates rupture of the lateral collateral ligament (Fig. 11).

Transverse Fracture of Lateral Malleolus

Transverse fracture of the lateral malleolus indicates that the avulsive force has been expended on the fracture and that there is no injury to the lateral collateral ligament. The fracture is associated with considerable soft-tissue swelling over the malleolus (Fig. 12).

EVERSION INJURIES

With forceful eversion of the foot, avulsive forces occur on the medial structures of the ankle and impacting forces on the lateral structures. Medial structural injuries of eversion consist of one of the following: (1) sprain of the

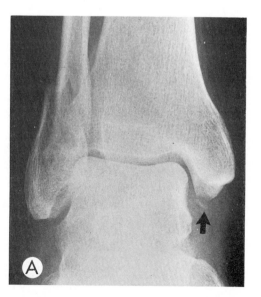

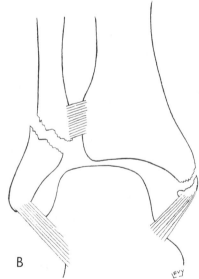

Fig. 14. Eversion injury of the ankle. There is an oblique fracture of the lateral malleolus indicating the eversion mechanism. The tibiofibular ligament is spared with the oblique fracture. A chip fracture is noted at the distal end of the medial malleolus, indicating avulsion of the deltoid ligament (arrow). (A) AP roentgenogram; (B) diagram.

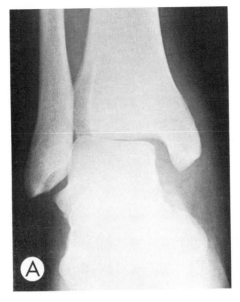
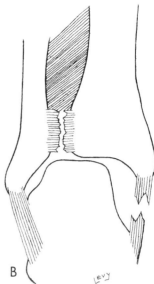

Fig. 15. Eversion injury of the ankle. No fracture is present. The talus is shifted laterally. In the absence of a spiral fracture of the fibula, this indicates tear of the tibiofibular and the medial collateral ligaments. (A) AP roentgenogram; (B) diagram of injury.

medial collateral (deltoid) ligament; (2) avulsion of the medial collateral ligament; (3) rupture of the medial collateral ligament; (4) transverse fracture of the medial malleolus (Fig. 13).

Lateral structural damage caused by talar dislocation includes the following: (1) oblique or spiral fracture of the lateral malleolus (Fig. 14); (2) tibiofibular ligament rupture with tibiofibular diastasis, without fracture of the fibula (Fig. 15); (3) tibiofibular ligament rupture with fracture of the fibula (Figs. 16 and 17).

Sprain of Medial Collateral Ligament

Sprain of the medial collateral ligament indicates rupture of some of the fibers, but the continuity of the ligament is intact. The roentgenogram shows only soft-tissue swelling distal to the medial malleolus. Abduction stress films are indicated to exclude a complete rupture.

Avulsion of Medial Collateral Ligament

Avulsion of the medial collateral ligament indicates that the ligament has been pulled from

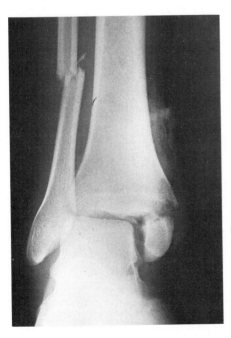
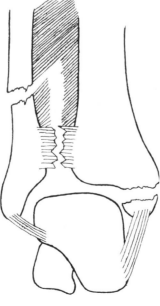

Fig. 16. Eversion injury of the ankle. The transverse fracture of the medial malleolus indicates the mechanism of the injury. There is lateral dislocation of the talus and a fracture of the fibula above the tibiofibular ligament attachment. This indicates a tibiofibular ligament tear. (A) AP roentgenogram; (B) diagram.

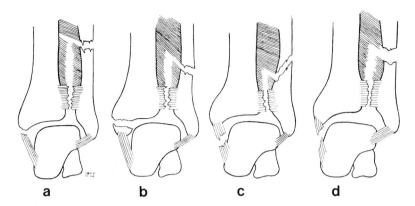

a   b   c   d

Fig. 17.   Eversion injuries with fracture above the tibiofibular joint. Avulsion of the deltoid ligament with tibiofibular ligament rupture accompanies the fracture. Note that the interosseous membrane is torn to the level of the fracture. (a) High fracture of the fibula; (b) transverse fracture of the medial malleolus with rupture of the tibiofibular ligament and fracture of the fibula (c); rupture of the body of the deltoid ligament with oblique fracture of the fibula and tear of the tibiofibular ligament; (d) rupture of the body of the deltoid ligament with tear of the tibiofibular ligament and transverse fracture of the fibula above the tibiofibular ligament.

its attachment to the medial malleolus. If small chips of bone accompany the avulsion, stress films are unnecessary, since the nature of the injury is clear. If there are no fractures, then stress films are indicated. The soft-tissue swelling lies at the level of the medial malleolus.

Rupture of Medial Collateral Ligament

Rupture of the medial collateral ligament occurs in the body of the ligament away from the bony attachment, and there will be no "sprain" fracture. Soft-tissue swelling is most prominent distal to the tip of the malleolus, and the same features are present as in a sprain. Abduction stress films are required to identify the injury. If the injury is associated with a spiral or oblique fracture of the distal fibula, diastasis of the

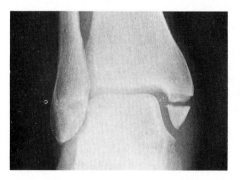

Fig. 18.   Transverse fracture of the medial malleolus. This indicates an eversion mechanism. The avulsion force has spared the medial collateral ligament. If multiple views fail to show evidence of a spiral fracture of the fibula, there must be a tibiofibular ligament tear. There is slight lateral dislocation of the talus.

tibiofibular joint, or fracture of the fibula above the tibiofibular ligament, a deltoid rupture must be present, and stress films are therefore unnecessary.

Transverse Fracture of Medial Malleolus

Transverse fracture of the medial malleolus indicates that the avulsion or eversion force was expended on the fracture, and thus medial collateral ligament injury is absent (Fig. 18).

Oblique Fracture of Lateral Malleolus

Oblique or spiral fracture of the lateral malleolus indicates the eversion mechanism. The fracture is due to the impact of the dislocated talus (Fig. 14). For the talus to dislocate and cause a spiral fracture, there must be rupture or avulsion of the medial collateral ligament or a transverse fracture of the medial malleolus. The spiral fracture of the tibia expends the impacting force, and the tibiofibular ligament will be intact, except perhaps for some of its fibers. Diastasis of the tibiofibular joint does not occur. The roentgenogram will show soft-tissue swelling in the region of the medial malleolus, with or without fractures, and soft-tissue swelling up to the level of the lateral malleolus, with spiral or oblique fracture. The tibiofibular joint is intact. Stress films are unnecessary.

Tibiofibular Ligament Rupture

Tibiofibular ligament rupture without fibular fracture may occur with an eversion injury when

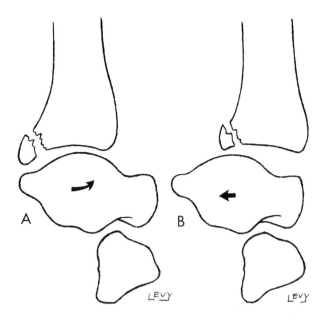

Fig. 19. Marginal posterior lip fracture of the tibia. This may be due either to inversion (A) or to posterior dislocation of the talus (B). It indicates a tear of the tibiofibular ligament.

the lateral malleolus is not fractured (Fig. 15). A chip fracture or a transverse fracture of the medial malleolus may be evident, but with medial collateral ligament tear, fracture of the medial malleolus does not occur. The roentgen features are soft-tissue swelling at or below the medial malleolus and soft-tissue swelling above the lateral malleolus as high as the midshaft of the fibula. Chip fracture or transverse fracture of the medial malleolus may be present. There may be dislocation of the talus and diastasis of the distal tibiofibular joint. *Eversion injuries may cause rupture of the deltoid and tibiofibular ligaments without fracture.* Talar dislocation and tibiofibular diastasis may not be apparent. The seriousness of the injury may be appreciated clinically and suspected roentgenographically from the sites of the soft-tissue swelling. Stress films may be indicated if no fracture, dislocation, or diastasis is identified.

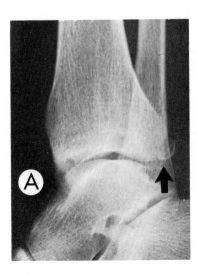

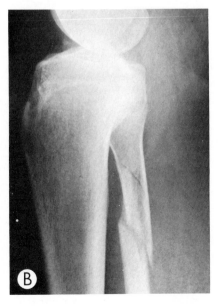

Fig. 20. Posterior lip fracture (arrow) with associated fracture of the proximal end of the fibula. When the tibiofibular ligament tears, a fracture of the fibular shaft must be suspected. (Courtesy of Dr. Norma Harris, Department of Radiology, Ben Taub Hospital, Houston, Texas.)

Tibiofibular Ligament Rupture With Fracture of Fibula Above Tibiofibular Ligament

Tibiofibular ligament rupture with fracture of the fibula above the tibiofibular ligament may be likened to the snapping of a twig. With a tear of the tibiofibular ligament and of the interosseous membrane, the fibula is abducted; the upper intact interosseous membrane fixes the proximal fibula, and the bone snaps like a twig. Fracture of the fibula more than 4 cm above the distal end indicates tibiofibular ligament tear with an eversion injury to the ankle (Fig. 16). The fracture may even occur in the proximal third of the fibula (Maisonneuve fracture), so that the radiograph in eversion injury must include the entire fibula.

Fracture of Posterior Margin of Distal Tibia

Fracture of the posterior margin of the distal tibia may involve only the lip or may incorporate up to 50% of the plafond.

Posterior marginal lip fractures may be caused by inversion injury or by posterior dislocation of the talus (Fig. 19). In the former, a small chip of bone is pulled from the posterolateral tibial surface, and in the latter a small chip of bone is separated from the middle portion of the posterior tibial surface by the dislocated talus. Whenever there is a chip fracture there must be widening of the mortise by either an oblique fracture of the lateral malleolus or a tear of the tibiofibular ligament. With inversion injury, the lip fracture follows displacement of the distal fibula. For this displacement to occur, the tibiofibular ligament must rupture or the lateral malleolus must fracture. If there is a tibiofibular ligament tear, a fracture of the shaft of the fibula may occur (Fig. 20).

The lip fracture due to posterior dislocation of the talus also indicates mortise widening because the ankle joint is narrower posteriorly. For the talus to dislocate posteriorly, the mortise must be widened, and either a fracture of the lateral malleolus or tear of the tibiofibular ligament must occur. The talus may be dislocated posteriorly without a lip fracture, but widening of the mortise must occur.

Larger fractures of the posterior tibia are usually vertical and may incorporate as much as 50% of the plafond. They are caused by a

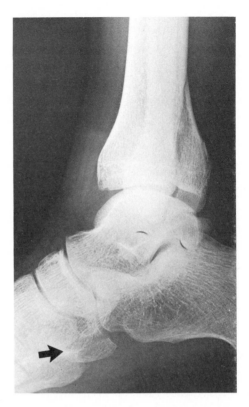

Fig. 21.   Large posterior tibial lip fracture. When the fragment is this large, the fracture is usually from a compressive force, and dislocation of the talus need not occur. The fracture of the cuboid (arrow) indicates the compressive mechanism.

compressive force with the foot in plantar flexion. Talar dislocation does not usually occur. There is often associated transverse or vertical fracture of the tarsal cuboid (Fig. 21). The amount of plafond incorporated in the fracture must be reported, for if it is over 25% to 30%, open fixation is usually indicated.

Small compression fractures of the talar articular surface indicate severe ankle injury. They may be particularly difficult to demonstrate. Almost perfect contour restoration and adequate immobilization are necessary to prevent secondary osteoarthritis.

Traumatic arthritis occurs in approximately 30% of ankle fractures, regardless of the treatment.[1,2,4,5] It may be the result of inaccurate reduction of the mortise or comminution of the plafond.[3] The arthritis may appear within a few months of the initial injury and is evidenced by joint space narrowing due to cartilage destruction.

REFERENCES

1. Burwell, HN, Charnley, AD: The treatment of displaced fractures at the ankle by rigid internal fixation and early joint movement. J Bone Joint Surg [Br] 47:634–660, 1965

2. Klossner O: Late results of operative and non-operative treatment of severe ankle fractures. Acta Chir Scand [Suppl] 293:1–93, 1962

3. Rockwood CA Jr, Green DP (eds): Fractures, vol 2. Philadelphia, Lippincott, 1975

4. Vasli S: Operative treatment of ankle fractures. Acta Chir Scand [Suppl] 226:1–74, 1957

5. Wilson, FC, Skilbred LA: Long-term results in the treatment of displaced bimalleolar fractures. J Bone Joint Surg [Am] 48:1065–1078, 1966

Foot

Lee F. Rogers and Robert E. Campbell

THE TOPIC of this article might be considered pedestrian; it certainly lacks charisma. Despite this obvious deficiency, it must be admitted that foot trauma is quite common. Fractures of the bones of the feet account for approximately 10% of all fractures, and they are encountered daily in the radiology department.

Bone and joint injuries can occur as a result of direct trauma, from objects falling on the foot, from falls, or from movement of the foot against a variety of objects. Injuries also occur from indirect trauma mediated either through tendon or capsular avulsion or through excessive torsional motion of a joint. In addition, overuse or unaccustomed activity may result in stress fracture.

ANATOMY

Traditionally the foot is divided into three anatomic parts:[12] the forefoot, consisting of the metatarsals and phalanges; the hindfoot, consisting of the talus and calcaneus; and the midfoot, consisting of the three cuneiform bones and the cuboid and navicular. Because of the large number of bones in close proximity, oblique projections are mandatory to properly display the various individual components to advantage. Thus, in addition to the standard AP and lateral views, oblique projections are required to fully evaluate injuries of the foot.

There are numerous accessory centers of ossification, sesamoid bones, and a few apophyseal growth centers that may be confused with fractures. The os trigonum, os tibiale externum, os peroneum, and os vesalianum are particularly common. The os supratalare and os supranaviculare are less common, but they may easily be mistaken for small avulsion fractures. The calcaneal apophysis, on the posterior margin of the os calcis, although denser than the parent bone and often normally fragmented, should not present a problem. However, the apophysis at the lateral margin of the base of the fifth metatarsal is easily mistaken for an avulsion fracture in a child or adolescent. This apophysis may be bipartite. Sesamoids of the great toe frequently arise from two or more centers that fail to unite. The epiphysis of the proximal phalanx of the great toe is at times bifid and may resemble an epiphyseal fracture. The epiphysis of the distal phalanges may be triangular in outline. In general, all of these variants can readily be distinguished from fractures by observing their intact smooth cortical surface as well as that of the adjacent apposed osseous structure, in contradistinction to the irregular surface and absence of cortical bone along the margins of a fracture. If you are unable to make this distinction, refer to the excellent demonstrations of these centers in standard texts,[19,23] obtain a comparative examination of the opposite side (since such variants are frequently bilateral), or examine the patient to determine if the pain and tenderness are related to the area in question. One of these steps should resolve the problem.

Motion of the foot is relatively complex, and the terminology used to designate these motions is complicated. *Plantar flexion* is motion toward the plantar surface of the foot; *dorsiflexion* is the opposite. The complex movements of *inversion* and *eversion* refer to changes in position and form of the whole foot when the foot is off the ground. Inversion is an inward rotation of the foot, and eversion is an outward rotation of the foot about its long axis. *Adduction* is inward rotation, and *abduction* is external rotation about the vertical axis. All of the above are sometimes considered as isolated movements, but they cannot occur independently. Inversion is usually associated with plantar flexion of the ankle joint, and eversion with dorsiflexion. The terms *pronation* and *supination* of the foot should be used only when the foot is bearing weight. Pronation refers to a downward rotation

Lee F. Rogers, M.D.: *Professor and Chairman, Department of Radiology, Northwestern University Medical School, Chicago, Ill.* Robert E. Campbell, M.D.: *Clinical Professor of Radiology, University of Pennsylvania School of Medicine; Deputy Director, Department of Radiology, Pennsylvania Hospital, Philadelphia, Pa.*

Reprint requests should be addressed to Dr. Lee F. Rogers, Department of Radiology, Northwestern University Medical School, 303 East Chicago Avenue, Chicago, Ill. 60611.

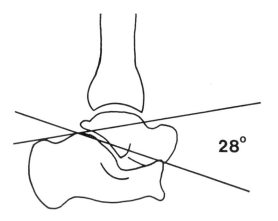

BOEHLER'S ANGLE
(20°–40°)

Fig. 1. Boehler angle. A line is drawn from the superior posterior margin of the tuberosity through the tip of the posterior facet. A second line is drawn from the tip of the posterior facet through the superior margin of the anterior process of the calcaneus. The normal angle is 20–40 degrees.

of the medial border of the foot and great toe toward the ground, and supination is the reverse movement that brings the lateral border of the foot into more direct contact with the ground.

CALCANEUS

The calcaneus is the largest tarsal bone, and it serves two principal functions: to bear weight

and to serve as a springboard for locomotion.[14] The large bony projection posterior to the talocalcaneal joint is referred to as the tuberosity. A platform of bone arising from the medial surface of the calcaneus, termed the sustentaculum tali, supports the anterior portion of the talus. The principal subtalar joint is formed in the midportion of the calcaneus on the posterior facet. The posterior facet is sloped so that its face projects anteriorly and superiorly. The anterior and medial facets of the talocalcaneal joint are found on the sustentaculum tali. The anterior process of the calcaneus and the posterior facet form an angle of approximately 100 degrees. The lateral portion of the talus, or tuber, sits within this angle. This is sometimes referred to as the tuber or crucial angle of the calcaneus.

The Boehler angle is useful in evaluation of calcaneal injuries (Fig. 1). This angle is formed by a line drawn on the lateral view of the foot from the superior posterior margin of the tuberosity through the superior tip of the posterior facet. A second line is drawn from the superior tip of the posterior facet through the superior margin of the anterior process of the calcaneus. Normally the Boehler angle measures 20 to 40 degrees.

Nonavulsion fracture of the os calcis is most commonly the result of falling from a height.

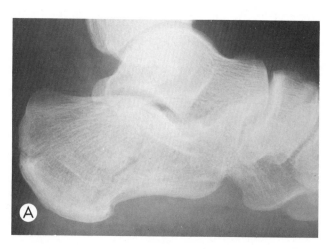

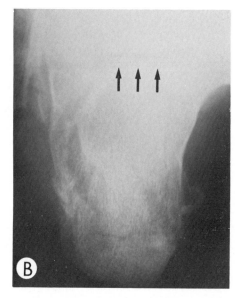

Fig. 2. Compressed comminuted fracture of the calcaneus: (A) Lateral view. The posterior facet is depressed. Boehler angle is 0 degrees. Fracture lines are apparent in the tuberosity. (B) Axial view. Numerous fracture lines are present, some extending into the posterior facet (arrows). The tuberosity is widened.

Approximately 10% of these fractures are bilateral, and a similar percentage are associated with vertebral body compression or posterior element fracture of the thoracolumbar spine.[22,27] It behooves the physician to know about these associated injuries, since they are well known to many alert plaintiff lawyers.

Complete radiographic examination of suspected calcaneal injuries requires AP, lateral, and internal oblique views of the foot, AP, internal, and external oblique views of the ankle, and an axial view of the calcaneus.[12] The oblique views of the ankle are very useful in demonstrating the posterior talocalcaneal articulation. The axial view should demonstrate the sustentaculum tali as well as the posterior talocalcaneal articulation. Multiple axial projections between 20 and 40 degrees may be necessary to accomplish this.

The critical determination in fractures of the calcaneus is whether or not the fracture line involves the subtalar joint and, if so, the degree of depression of the posterior facet.[10] Approximately three-fourths of all nonavulsion fractures of the calcaneus involve the subtalar joint, and three-fourths of these are associated with depression.

Crushing injuries result in comminuted fractures with depression of the central and lateral fragments of the posterior facet. It is important to determine the Boehler angle to assess the amount of depression of the posterior facet of the talocalcaneal joint (Fig. 2). A Boehler angle of less than 20 degrees indicates depression. At times the compression is severe, and the rotation of the calcaneal fragment is such that the subtalar joint becomes incongruous. This is an important observation. Vertical fractures may extend into the subtalar joint without compression (Fig. 3).

Those fractures that spare the subtalar joint are usually of the avulsion type. They involve the sustentaculum tali, the anterior process in the region of calcaneocuboid (Fig. 7) and calcaneonavicular joints, the superior portion of the tuberosity (beak fracture, representing avulsion by a portion of the Achilles tendon), and the medial or lateral surface of the tuberosity.[20,22] Vertical fracture of the tuberosity frequently extends obliquely from the medial to the lateral surface of the calcaneus and may very easily be overlooked on the lateral view. The axial view is

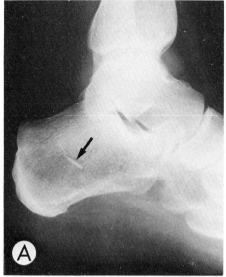

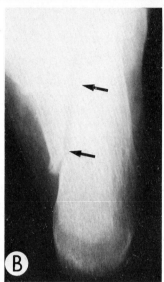

Fig. 3.   Linear vertical fracture of calcaneus: (A) Fracture line is difficult to visualize on the lateral projection (arrow). (B) It is readily apparent on the axial projection (arrows).

necessary to clearly demonstrate the fracture line (Fig. 3).

Stress fracture occurs in the tuberosity of the calcaneus.[9,26] It commonly results from running or unaccustomed long-distance hiking. As with other stress fractures, it is not immediately evident, but appears about 10 days to several months after the exertional episode. It is manifest by an ill-defined line of sclerosis within the tuberosity, paralleling the posterior margin of the calcaneus (Fig. 4). The sclerotic line represents endosteal callus formation.

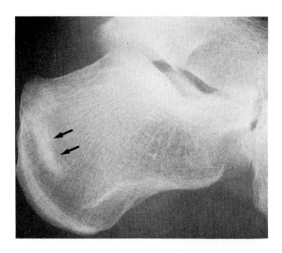

Fig. 4. Stress fracture. Note the ill-defined area of scle-rosis (arrows) parallel to the posterior cortex of the calcaneus. The film was obtained 14 days after onset of symptoms.

TALUS

The talus is the second most common site of fracture of the tarsal bones. Approximately 60% of the surface of the talus is covered by articular cartilage. Its blood supply is tenuous, and it is therefore susceptible to aseptic ne-crosis.[12,21] Furthermore, it is the only bone in the lower extremity without muscle attach-ments, being connected to adjacent structures only by articular capsule, synovial membranes, and ligamentous attachments, so that disloca-tion is frequent.[3]

The most common talar fractures are the chip and avulsion variety.[21] These occur at four main sites, the superior surface of the neck and head, and the lateral, medial, and posterior aspects of the body. The most common is the anterosuperior surface of the neck at the point

of attachment of the ankle joint. Fracture of the lateral aspect of the body of the talus involves the posterior articular facet where it projects laterally beneath the tip of the lateral malleolus. The deep fibers of the deltoid ligament are at-tached on the medial surface of the body just below and behind the tip of the medial malleolus. Avulsion fracture may occur at this point. Fracture of the posterior talar surface in-volves the posterior tubercle. In severe plantar flexion the posterior talar tubercle may become wedged between the calcaneus and the posterior rim of the tibia and sustain a fracture. This frac-ture must be differentiated from the accessory center of ossification at this site, the os trigonum.

The second most common talar injury is vertical fracture of the neck (Fig. 5B).[15] This may occur with or without dislocation of the body of the talus. The mechanism is usually a force from below that drives the neck of the talus upward against the anterior lip of the tibia. This mechanism was initially identified in World War I aviators and thus was designated as avia-tor's fracture or aviator's astragalus.[5] The frac-ture occurred when pilots crash-landed and the rudder bar was jammed against the sole of the foot. Today these fractures are seen following head-on automobile collision. Since the blood supply of the talus, much like that of the carpo-navicular, is tenuous, aseptic necrosis of the proximal fragment often occurs in vertical frac-ture of the neck, despite healing of the fracture.

If the dorsiflexion force continues after the neck is fractured and the body of the talus be-comes locked in the ankle mortice, then the re-mainder of the foot may continue forward to produce a subtalar dislocation.[3] In addition,

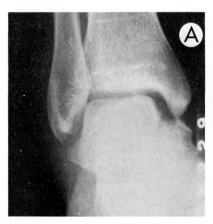
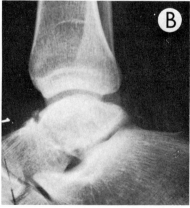

Fig. 5. Vertical fracture of the neck of the talus with medial subtalar dislocation: (A) AP view reveals medial disloca-tion of the foot. The talus remains in the ankle mortice. (B) Lateral view demonstrates the fracture of the neck of the talus. The subtalar dislocation is difficult to identify in this view.

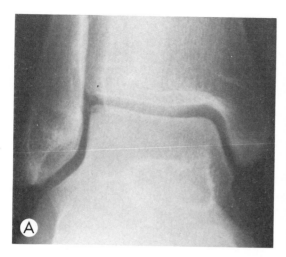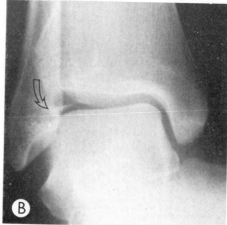

Fig. 6. Osteochondral fracture of the dome of the talus: (A) AP view. There is only a suggestion of irregularity of the superior lateral aspect of the talus. (B) Inversion stress view reveals an osteochondral fracture of the dome of the talus (arrow) and altered joint mortice.

fracture of the neck may be associated with posterior dislocation of the body of the talus. The mechanism of injury is continuation of the dorsiflexion force that produced the fracture of the neck and then a rupture of ligamentous structures that bind the talus to the calcaneus and tibia. The body of the talus is then forced backward out of the ankle mortice. The posterior dislocation of the proximal fragment may be minimal and often is overlooked by the radiologist. This can be a serious omission, since the morbidity associated with an unreduced dislocation is great.

Probably the most disabling and fortunately the least frequent injury of the talus is total dislocation occurring as a result of complete disruption of the ankle and subtalar joints. This is usually an open injury, and it may be associated with fracture of the neck of the talus.

Subtalar dislocation of the foot consists of simultaneous dislocations of the talonavicular joint and the talocalcaneal joint. They occur more commonly medially than laterally (Fig. 5). The medial dislocation has been reported in basketball players who land on an inverted foot after leaping upward for the ball.[13]

Osteochondral fractures occur at the dome of the talus as a result of inversion or eversion injuries at the ankle.[2,7] As a result of tilting of the talus within the ankle mortice, an osteochondral fragment is avulsed when the apposing surface of the talus encounters the medial or lateral malleolus. The resultant fracture consists of a fragment of bone at either the superior medial or superior lateral margin of the talus. Frequently these fragments are small and can only be identified on inversion and eversion stress films (Fig. 6). Such fractures are commonly mistaken for osteochondritis dissecans.

NAVICULAR BONE

Fractures of the navicular bone are relatively uncommon.[6,8,12] The most frequent is an avulsion fracture of the dorsal surface of the talonavicular joint, often identified only in the true lateral projection. Next in frequency is fracture involving the tuberosity on the medial aspect of the navicular bone (Fig. 7). The tuberosity serves as the major insertion for the posterior tibial tendon. This fracture results from acute eversion of the foot, which places increased tension on the posterior tibial tendon. Characteristically the fracture is not displaced because the other insertions of the tendon on the plantar surface of the foot maintain position. The fracture may therefore be difficult to visualize. Care must be taken to differentiate a fracture of the navicular tuberosity from the accessory center of ossification, the os tibial externum, which lies just posterior to the tuberosity. Fracture of the tuberosity is at times associated with fracture of the cuboid bone. Fracture of the body of the navicular bone may occur in either the horizontal or vertical plane and may be associated with navicular dislocation.

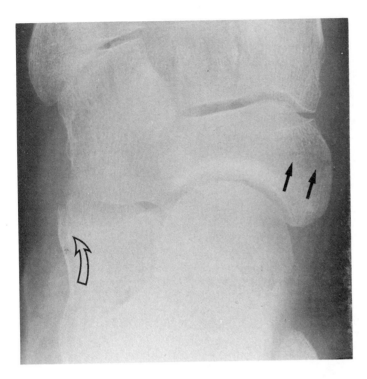

Fig. 7. Fracture of the medial tuberosity of the navicular (straight arrows) and anterior process of the calcaneus (curved arrow).

CUBOID AND CUNEIFORMS

Isolated fractures of the cuboid are rare.[6,12] Avulsion fractures may occur from direct trauma, particularly laterally. These must be differentiated from the accessory centers of ossification, the os peroneum (a sesamoid bone in the peroneus longus tendon that is occasionally bipartite) and the os vesalianum. Compression fracture of the cuboid or anterior process of the calcaneus is associated with fracture of the tuberosity of the navicular bone.[16]

Isolated fractures of the cuneiforms are most unusual. Fractures of the distal margin of the cuneiforms and cuboid bone are usually associated with dislocation of the tarsometatarsal joint. Therefore, if such a fracture is identified, you are obligated to exclude the possibility of an associated tarsometatarsal dislocation.

TARSOMETATARSAL FRACTURE DISLOCATION (LISFRANC)

The tarsometatarsal fracture dislocation is commonly referred to as the Lisfranc dislocation, although this injury was not described by him.[4] Lisfranc was a surgeon in Napoleon's armies who described an amputation procedure through the tarsometatarsal joints.

Strong ligaments attach the cuneiforms and the cuboid to the bases of the metatarsals.[1] The base of the second metatarsal is recessed from the normal curvilinear plane of the tarsometatarsal joints. This recess is created by the relatively short middle cuneiform. Thus the base of the second metatarsal is locked between the medial and lateral cuneiforms. There is considerable soft-tissue support on the plantar surface of the tarsometatarsal joints, whereas these joints are supported only by ligamentous structures on their dorsal surfaces.

The Lisfranc injury is basically a dorsal dislocation of the tarsometatarsal joints that may be produced by a fall from a height, by falling down a flight of stairs, or simply by stepping off a curb.[24,25] Usually the metatarsal heads are fixed on the ground, and the weight of the body forces the hindfoot down against the base of the metatarsals in association with some degree of rotation. These abnormal forces result in disruption of the ligaments about the tarsometatarsal joints and dorsal dislocation of the metatarsals. Another mechanism is for the body to rotate around the fixed forefoot, such as might occur when falling from a horse with the foot remaining in the stirrup.

There are two basic forms of injury (Fig. 8).[24] The homolateral type is a dislocation of the

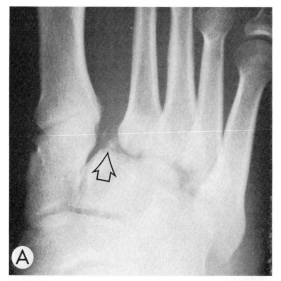

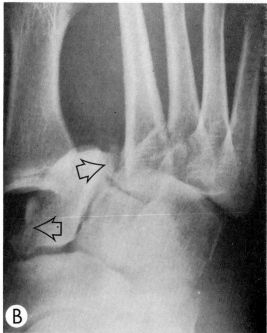

Fig. 8. Lisfranc dislocation of the tarsal-metatarsal joints: (A) Homolateral type. The second through fifth metatarsals are dislocated laterally. Note the associated fractures at the base of the second metatarsal (arrows). (B) Divergent type. The second through fifth metatarsals are dislocated laterally and the first metatarsal medially. There are associated fractures (arrows) of the first cuneiform and base of the second metatarsal.

metatarsals, usually four or all five, more commonly lateral than medial (Fig. 8A). The second is the divergent type wherein there is later displacement of the second through fifth metatarsals and medial displacement of the first

metatarsal. The mechanism of the latter is complex. The most common fractures associated with these dislocations are transverse fracture at the base of the recessed second metatarsal, compression or chip fracture of the distal margin of the cuboid bone, and chip fractures of the base of the metatarsals and adjacent tarsal bones.[11] Fractures of the shafts of the second, third, and fourth metatarsals occur less commonly. In the divergent type there may be dislocation between the middle and medial cuneiform-navicular joints or a fracture of the navicular bone.

The medial aspect of the second metatarsal and the medial aspect of the middle cuneiform should always be in line. When this alignment is disrupted or when there is a fracture of the base of the second metatarsal or a compression or chip fracture of the distal margin of the cuboid bone, it is very likely that a tarsometatarsal dislocation exists. The appearances of the metatarsal-cuneiform and metatarsal-cuboid articulations are highly variable, depending on radiographic projection. Comparison views of the opposite foot may be necessary to clarify or identify the injury.

FRACTURES OF METATARSALS AND PHALANGES

Fractures of the shaft and neck of the metatarsals and of the phalanges are usually the result of heavy objects falling on the foot.[28] Less commonly, the phalanges may be fractured as the foot strikes furniture or other objects during walking, particularly in the dark. These fractures may be transverse (Figs. 9A and B), oblique, or comminuted. Epiphyseal injuries can occur in the adolescent at either the head of a metatarsal, or the base of the first metatarsal or a phalanx (Fig. 9C). These are either Salter-Harris type 1 or type 2 and carry a favorable prognosis. On occasion, the epiphysis of the distal phalanx of the great toe arises from two ossification centers (Fig. 9D).[18] This is easily mistaken for an epiphyseal fracture. In addition, Freiberg disease (avascular necrosis of the head of the second metatarsal) and subarticular osteolysis of a metatarsal head or base of a proximal phalanx in diabetic osteopathy should not be confused with fracture.

One of the more frequent injuries of the foot is transverse fracture at the base of the fifth

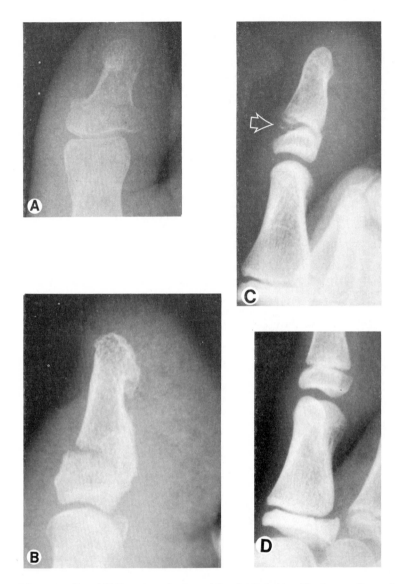

Fig. 9.   Phalangeal fractures: (A and B) Transverse fracture of the distal phalanx. The fracture is not clearly seen in the AP view. (C) Epiphyseal injury. The growth plate is widened, and a small metaphyseal fragment (arrow) is demonstrated. (D) Bipartite epiphysis of the proximal phalanx of the great toe. A normal variant, not a fracture.

metatarsal (Fig. 10A).[17,28] This is the result of a plantar flexion and inversion injury of the foot that may be sustained by stepping off a curb or by falling when walking on stairs. This is actually an avulsion injury mediated through the peroneus brevis tendon, which is attached to the base of the fifth metatarsal. The fracture fragment may be confused with the apophysis of the fifth metatarsal in children; however, the apophysis is longitudinally oriented at the lateral aspect of the base of the fifth metatarsal, as opposed to the transverse orientation of the fracture (Fig. 10B).

There are also two accessory centers of ossification in this area that may be mistaken for this fracture. These are the os vesalianum, occurring just proximal to the base of the fifth metatarsal, and the os peroneum, a sesamoid bone lying within the peroneus tendon at the lateral margin of the cuboid bone. The original description of this fracture was by Sir Robert Jones,[17] who reported a fracture at the base of the fifth metatarsal that he had sustained while dancing. Thus this fracture is sometimes known as the Jones fracture or dancer's fracture. Clinically it is easily mistaken for fracture of the

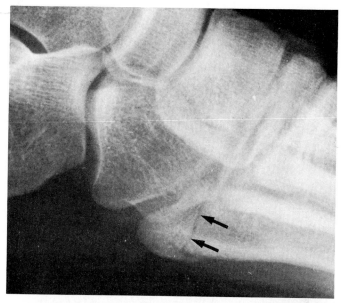

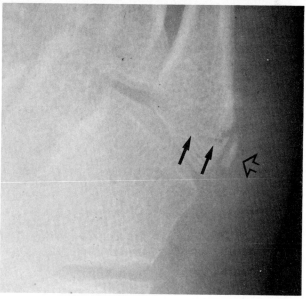

Fig. 10. Jones fracture of base of the fifth metatarsal: (A) An undisplaced transverse fracture (arrow) in an adult. (B) A similar transverse fracture (solid arrows) in an 11-year-old. Note the longitudinally oriented apophysis (open arrow) at the base of the fifth metatarsal.

lateral malleolus because of swelling over the lateral aspect of the ankle. The clinician may then order only a roentgenographic examination of the ankle. Care should always be taken to include the base of the fifth metatarsal on the lateral roentgenogram of the ankle and to look specifically at this area for this common fracture.

The metatarsals are also the site of the most common stress fracture, the "march" fracture of the second, third, or (rarely) fourth metatarsal.[9,26] It is particularly common in the military recruit population, but it can be en-

countered in all walks of life. (Isn't that outrageous!) As a step or stride is initiated, the load applied to the forefoot places maximum force on the head of the second metatarsal or, in some individuals, on the third metatarsal. With increased stress, there is a physiologic response of increased osteoclastic activity, microinfractions of bone, and finally a frank fracture in the metatarsal shaft, usually distally. The radiographic findings often are not initially evident. In 7 to 10 days a transverse radiolucency appears, indicating a site of fracture, and is followed by fluffy periosteal reaction about

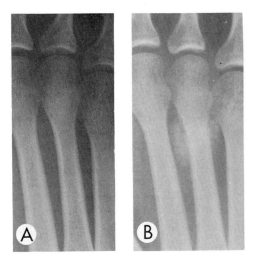

Fig. 11. Stress fracture of a metatarsal: (A) Film made 3 days after onset of symptoms is normal. (B) Fluffy periosteal callus is present about the distal shaft of the third metatarsal 3 weeks later.

the fracture site (Fig. 11). At times this periosteal new bone is extensive. Uncommonly, a stress fracture appears at the base of the first metatarsal. This is of the endosteal variety, similar to that seen in the calcaneus, and thus it presents as a line of dense bone traversing the base of the first metatarsal.

SESAMOIDS

Occasionally there is a transverse fracture of one of the sesamoids of the great toe, more commonly the tibial sesamoid. This has been described in ballet dancers, in whom it may actually represent a stress fracture. It must be remembered that the sesamoids may be bipartite or may arise from several centers of ossification.[19,28] These should not be mistaken for fracture. This may be difficult, since the fracture fragments are not necessarily widely distracted.

REFERENCES

1. Aitken AP, Poulson D: Dislocations of the tarsometatarsal joint. J Bone Joint Surg [Am] 45:246–260, 1963

2. Berndt AL, Harty M: Transchondral fractures (osteochondritis dissecans) of the talus. J Bone Joint Surg [Am] 41:988–1020, 1959

3. Buckingham WW Jr, LeFlore I: Subtalar dislocation of the foot. J Trauma 13:753–765, 1973

4. Cassebaum WH: Lisfranc fracture-dislocations. Clin Orthop 30:116–129, 1963

5. Coltart WD: "Aviator's astragalus." J Bone Joint Surg [Br] 34:545–566, 1952

6. Crenshaw AH: Campbell's Operative Orthopaedics, vol. 2 (ed 4). St Louis, CV Mosby, 1963

7. Davidson AM, Steele HD, MacKenzie DA, et al: A review of twenty-one cases of transchondral fracture of the talus. J Trauma 7:378–415, 1967

8. Day AJ: The treatment of injuries to the tarsal navicular. J Bone Joint Surg 29:359–366, 1947

9. Devas M: Stress Fractures. London, Churchill-Livingstone, 1975, pp 148–173

10. Essex-Lopresti P: Fractures of the os calcis: The mechanism, reduction technique, and results in fractures of the os calcis. Br J Surg 39:395–419, 1952

11. Foster SC, Foster RR: Lisfranc's tarsometatarsal fracture-dislocation. Radiology 120:79–83, 1976

12. Giannestras NJ, Sammarco GJ: Fractures and dislocations in the foot, in Rockwood CA and Green DP (eds): Fractures, vol. 2, Philadelphia, JB Lippincott, 1975, p 1400

13. Grantham SA: Medial subtalar dislocation: Five cases with a common etiology. J Trauma 4:845–849, 1964

14. Harty M: Anatomic considerations in injuries of the calcaneus. Orthop Clin North Am 4:179–183, 1973

15. Hawkins LG: Fractures of the neck of the talus. J Bone Joint Surg [Am] 52:991–1002, 1970

16. Hermel MB, Gershon-Cohen J: The nutcracker fracture of the cuboid by indirect violence. Radiology 60:850–854, 1953

17. Jones R: Fracture of the base of the fifth metatarsal bone by indirect violence. Ann Surg 35:697–700, 1902

18. Keats TE: An Atlas of Normal Roentgen Variants That May Simulate Disease. Chicago, Year Book, 1973, p 215

19. Koehler A, Zimmer EA: Borderlands of the Normal and Early Pathologic in Skeletal Roentgenology (ed 11). New York, Grune & Stratton, 1968, pp 466–467

20. Lance EM, Carey EJ, Wade PA: Fractures of the os calcis: A follow-up study. J Trauma 4:15–56, 1964

21. Pennal GF: Fractures of the talus. Clin Orthop 30:53–63, 1963

22. Rowe CR, Sakellarides T, Freeman PA, et al: Fractures of the os calcis. JAMA 184:98–101, 1963

23. Shultz RJ: The Language of Fracture. Baltimore, Williams & Wilkins, 1972, pp 120–164

24. Wiley JJ: The mechanism of tarso-metatarsal joint injuries. J Bone Joint Surg [Br] 53:474–482, 1971

25. Wilson DW: Injuries of the tarso-metatarsal joints. Etiology, classification and results of treatment. J Bone Joint Surg [Br] 54:677–686, 1972

26. Wilson ES, Katz FN: Stress fractures. An analysis of 250 consecutive cases. Radiology 92:481–486, 1969

27. Wilson JN: Watson-Jones Fractures and Joint Injuries, Vol. 2 (ed 5). London, Churchill-Livingstone, 1976, pp 1091–1211

28. Zatzkin HR: Trauma to the foot. Semin Roentgenol 5:419–435, 1970

Pediatric Fractures

FRACTURES in children involve good news and bad news. The good news is that repair is usually prompt, and growth and remodeling can correct even marked angular deformities. The bad news is that fractures that involve the growing epiphysis may result in progressive deformity. Thus it is important to identify the site and nature of the skeletal injury as accurately as possible. The anatomy and physiology of children's bones favor certain types of injury, such as greenstick fracture and epiphyseal separation. Furthermore, the healing pattern of a child's fracture may itself simulate disease.

ANATOMY AND PHYSIOLOGY

During the growth period, the long tubular bones are characterized by cartilaginous epiphyses containing centers of ossification at both ends of the diaphysis. The short tubular bones have an epiphysis at only one end of the bone. The blood supply to the diaphysis is via nutrient vessels and periosteal vessels; the epiphyses are supplied from vessels arising in the adjacent joint capsules. Only in early life do minute branches of the diaphyseal vessels extend from the metaphysis into the epiphysis. Thus, growth cartilage of the epiphysis is not supplied by vessels on the metaphyseal side of the zone of provisional calcification, but by vessels on the side on which the ossification center makes its appearance and enlarges[16] (Fig. 1).

Periosteal attachments to the shaft are less firm than in adults; the most firm are the terminal attachments to the epiphysis surrounding the cartilage-shaft junction. The intraarticular margins of the radiologically invisible cartilaginous epiphyses persist as articular cartilage after the ossification center attains its maximal size; the growth cartilage is obliterated when the epiphyses unite with the shaft.

PRINCIPLES OF RADIOGRAPHIC EXAMINATION[19]

The best possible films should, of course, be obtained, but elegance of photographic demonstration should not take precedence over the patient's comfort and safety. Radiographic examination should be undertaken only after the child has been seen by a physician and there is assurance that shock and significant hemorrhage are absent and that movement and delay in management are not likely to have an adverse effect.

The projections should be at right angles to each other, preferably frontal and lateral views. If the patient cannot be optimally positioned, films at any incidence can be obtained, but the second film should be at right angle to the first. Both the proximal and distal extremities of the bone examined should be included, if not on a single film, at least on two overlapping films taken at the same angle with no change in the position of the patient. Occasionally, nonroutine projections may be necessary to define the extent and nature of an injury, or even to detect the fracture when clinical signs are strong or soft-tissue changes suggest deep injury. On the initial examination, the uninjured side should also be examined in identical projections; these provide an individualized control that may solve problems of overdiagnosis and underdiagnosis.

TYPES OF FRACTURES

Diaphyseal Fracture

The garden variety of fracture in children is that of the shaft of a tubular bone. Healing is almost impossible to prevent. The statement has been made that union will occur so long as the fractured fragments are in the same extremity. In almost any fracture of the shaft of a tubular bone, healing and good realignment are favored by proximity of the injury to the end of the bone and younger age of the child.[5] Both of these factors are related to the amount and activity of potential for bone growth near the fracture site. Deformity in the plane of motion of the adjacent

Frederic N. Silverman, M.D.: *Professor of Clinical Radiology and Clinical Pediatrics, Department of Radiology, Stanford University School of Medicine, Stanford University Medical Center, Stanford, Calif.*

Reprint requests should be addressed to Dr. Frederic N. Silverman, Department of Radiology, Stanford University Medical Center, Stanford, Calif. 94305.

© *1978 by Grune & Stratton, Inc.*

0037-198X/78/1302-0010$0100/0

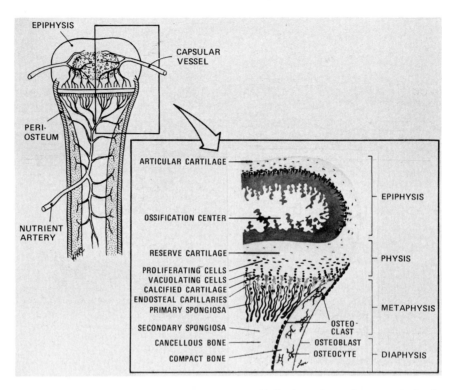

Fig. 1. Diagram of the blood supply of a long tubular bone in a child. The inset shows the anatomic detail at and near the growth plate of the epiphysis.

joint is more effectively corrected than deformity perpendicular to the plane of motion.[1] For example, anterior or posterior angulation of a supracondylar fracture of the humerus in a young child will result in very little deformity, whereas medial or lateral angulation may result in unsightly or disabling changes in the carrying angle.

Angulation and overriding deformities can correct spontaneously to an amazing degree, so that the radiologist's report should avoid implying that perfect approximation must be accomplished. Hyperemia in healing may actually cause overgrowth of the affected bone. In fractured femur, up to 1 cm of overriding can be spontaneously corrected. The villain in the piece is rotational deformity, and this is why the joints proximal and distal to the fracture must be shown. End-to-end approximation in a carefully coned film of the fracture site may miss the fact that one fragment is rotated in relation to the other, so that when healing is complete, the thigh may be facing forward while the knee faces medially or laterally. In these circumstances ambulation is difficult, to say the least.

The orthopedist is aware of this problem, but it does not hurt for the radiologist to call his attention to rotational deformity.

In the forearm and leg, films in two projections at right angles to each other may indicate excessive proximity of fractured elements of radius and ulna or tibia and fibula, respectively, that may lead to interosseous fusion during healing, with consequent loss of rotational functions. A subtle fracture at a different level in the companion bone should be sought when an obvious fracture is present. Associated dislocation of the otherwise unaffected bone should not be overlooked, as in Monteggia fracture, in which fracture of the ulna is associated with dislocation of the radial head.

Comminuted fractures are less common in children than in adults, probably because of the increased flexibility of young bones. With greater force, however, fragments of cortex may be separated from the major fragments, and if these are not incorporated in the healing callus, they may remain free and become symptomatic.[11]

The fracture site should be examined carefully for evidence of preexisting lesions that categorizes the fracture as pathologic. Bone cyst and fibrous dysplasia are common dysplastic precursors, but systemic dysplasias, inflammatory processes, and neoplasms may also predispose to fracture. Stress fractures occur in the upper third of the tibia, the lower half of the fibula,[9] and the metatarsals, and in other bones with less frequency. They are characterized by pain and tenderness at the site, with no history of antecedent injury. Local transverse bands of increased density, often with a central radiolucent stripe, and varying amounts of subperiosteal new bone formation extending proximally and distally are demonstrable.

Vascular damage may be a complication of any fracture, but in children the incidence is highest in supracondylar fracture of the elbow and in fracture of the distal third of the femur. A grossly displaced fracture and one with a sharp pointed end should be especially suspect.[17]

Greenstick Fracture

The relative elasticity of young bones may permit a bend to occur in which the cortex on only one side is disrupted. The affected bone bends like a green twig and remains bent. Because of frequent exaggeration of the deformity as the bone grows, a midshaft greenstick fracture is usually converted to a complete fracture and then positioned for immobilization and healing.

Acute bowing of forearm. Borden[2] recently described acute bowing of the forearm resulting from longitudinal stresses on the bone. Microfractures occur on the concave side of the bowed bone. Fracture of one bone of the forearm with acute bowing of the other is common. Comparison views of the unaffected limb are especially important because of the subtle nature of the findings (Fig. 2). The bowed bone is resistant to the usual orthopedic reduction and, in older children, may seriously limit pronation and supination on healing. Bowing differs from greenstick fracture in the extent of the curve, which blends imperceptibly into the bone at both ends, and in the absence of subperiosteal new bone during healing.[6] As with greenstick fracture, vigorous manipulation

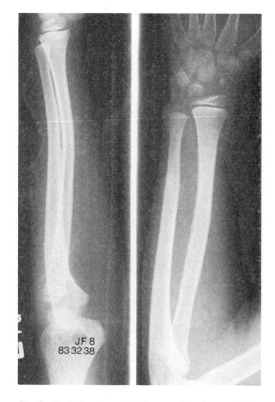

Fig. 2. Acute bowing of the bones of the forearm following longitudinal compression. The deformity is not visible in the AP projection but is obvious in the lateral. No fracture lines are visible. (Courtesy of Dr. R. H. Wilkinson, Boston.)

under general anesthesia to produce discontinuity of bone with appropriate realignment of the fragments may be necessary to prevent persistent deformity.

Torus (Buckling) Fracture

Injury insufficient to disrupt continuity of a bone may result in buckling of the cortex. This usually occurs at a site where more force would have produced an obvious fracture. The metaphysis of a bone is commonly involved because the cortex is thinnest in this region and thus less resistant to stress. Children with osteoporosis from any cause may also develop torus fracture (Fig. 3). Exquisite local tenderness in the area of injury may be the indication for oblique projections if the standard ones do not show the telltale break in the smooth course of the cortical bone. Although it is of little concern from the standpoint of deformity, torus fracture may be disturbingly symptomatic.[20] The term *torus* is derived from the vocabulary

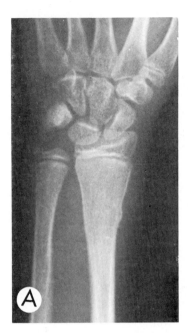
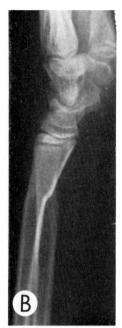

Fig. 3. Torus fracture of the radius: (A) AP view shows slight buckling of the radial cortex. Note the fracture of the ulnar styloid process. (B) Lateral view shows minimal angulation deformity.

of architecture, referring to the bulges on the base of a column.

Spiral Fracture of Tibia (Toddler Fracture)

An oblique fracture of the tibial shaft (toddler fracture) commonly occurs in children in their second or third year when falls or clumsiness in ambulation provide twisting forces that disrupt the bone. Displacement is minimal or absent because of the splinting effect on the intact fibula, so that an obvious fracture in one plane may be invisible in another (Fig. 4). The usual clinical evidence is that with no known injury the child refuses to bear weight on one leg, after having been normally active. The fracture usually heals without incident. The child restricts his activity until healing is well advanced. Many of these fractures go unrecognized.

Epiphyseal Fracture

The classification of epiphyseal injuries by Salter and Harris,[12] already alluded to in this symposium (p. 000), has achieved wide acceptance. Location of the fracture line has implications with respect to the mechanism of injury and to possible complications (Fig. 5). Salter-Harris type I fracture results from a horizontal shearing force separating the epiphysis from the shaft through the zone of calcification. Torsion or avulsion forces may do the same. The intact periosteum limits displacement of the epiphysis,

and none may be obvious initially. Subperiosteal hemorrhage lifts the periosteal envelope and probably stretches it, so that displacement may appear or increase prior to radiographic evidence of healing. Type I epiphyseal fracture is

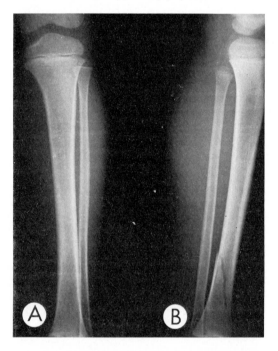

Fig. 4. Spiral fracture of tibia. The child refused to bear weight on the left leg. There had been no history of trauma. (A) AP projection is normal in spite of distinct tenderness over the distal fourth of the tibia. (B) The fracture is obvious in lateral projection.

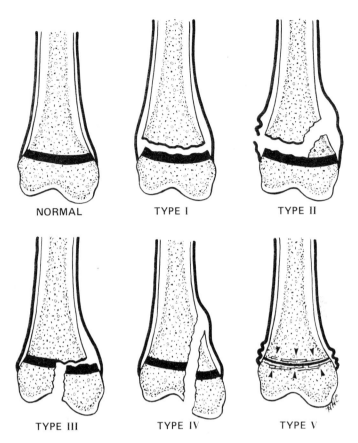

Fig. 5. Salter-Harris classification of epiphyseal fractures, modified from various sources.

NORMAL   TYPE I   TYPE II

TYPE III   TYPE IV   TYPE V

common in the distal radius; slipped femoral epiphysis is a special form of type 1 epiphyseal fracture, as is epiphyseal displacement in scurvy.

Significant early epiphyseal displacement signifies periosteal rupture and is associated with a detached fragment of the metaphysis. This is the type II epiphyseal fracture. It results from a lateral displacement force. Periosteal rupture is usually on the side opposite the metaphyseal fragment.

Recognition of type II fracture when the epiphysis is entirely or largely cartilaginous is facilitated by reference to the time of appearance of the secondary ossification centers[8] (Table 1). For example, a 5-year-old child with a cartilaginous epiphyseal separation at the elbow may present a small bone density in the region of the lateral epicondyle. No such center is seen on the control film of the healthy side, but asymmetry of appearance is not unusual. However, when note is made that the center for the lateral epicondyle appears on the average at about 11 years of age in boys, it becomes clear that there is a type II epiphyseal fracture and

that the bone density is not the center for the lateral epicondyle but is actually a fragment of avulsed bone.

Both types I and II epiphyseal fractures usually heal without sequelae when displacement is adequately reduced. Marked displacement of the head of the femur, however, may be followed by aseptic necrosis, since the blood supply comes largely, if not exclusively, from vessels on the surface of the intracapsular portion of the femoral neck.[16] These vessels may be disrupted completely by the displacement. An alternative explanation for the aseptic necrosis is mechanical injury to the femoral head accompanying the epiphyseal separation. Reconstitution of vascular supply probably occurs with sufficient speed and efficiency to make aseptic necrosis an uncommon complication.

Type III epiphyseal fracture consists of vertical fracture through the epiphysis continuous with the horizontal fracture through the calcified cartilage at the cartilage-shaft junction. A step-off of the articular margin of the ossification center may be the only clue. Careful restitution of the smooth joint surface is important

Table 1. Age-at-Appearance Percentiles for Major Postnatal Ossification Centers (in Years)*

	Percentiles					
	Boys			Girls		
Ossification Center	5th	50th	95th	5th	50th	95th
1. Head of humerus	—	.03	.32	—	.03	.30
2. Proximal epiphysis of tibia	—	.04	.10	—	.01	.04
3. Coracoid process of scapula	—	.04	.36	—	.03	.42
4. Cuboid of tarsus	—	.07	.30	—	.05	.16
5. Capitate of carpus	—	.25	.60	—	.15	.56
6. Hamate of carpus	.03	.31	.82	—	.18	.59
7. Capitulum of humerus	.06	.33	1.07	.05	.26	.77
8. Head of femur	.06	.35	.64	.04	.33	.62
9. Third cuneiform of tarsus	.05	.46	1.58	—	.23	1.23
10. Greater tubercle of humerus	.25	.83	2.33	.20	.51	1.14
11. Primary center, middle segment of 5th toe	—	1.04	3.81	—	.74	2.08
12. Distal epiphysis of radius	.53	1.10	2.30	.38	.82	1.70
13. Epiphysis, distal segment of 1st toe	.71	1.21	2.10	.39	.78	1.68
14. Epiphysis, middle segment of 4th toe	.40	1.21	2.88	.40	.92	3.00
15. Epiphysis, proximal segment of 3d finger	.77	1.37	2.15	.41	.85	1.61
16. Epiphysis, middle segment of 3d toe	.41	1.40	4.27	.21	1.02	2.47
17. Epiphysis, proximal segment of 2d finger	.78	1.41	2.17	.40	.87	1.64
18. Epiphysis, proximal segment of 4th finger	.80	1.49	2.40	.41	.90	1.66
19. Epiphysis, distal segment of 1st finger	.75	1.51	2.70	.42	.99	1.73
20. Epiphysis, proximal segment of 3d toe	.90	1.58	2.52	.51	1.05	1.88
21. Epiphysis of 2d metacarpal	.93	1.61	2.82	.64	1.09	1.69
22. Epiphysis, proximal segment of 4th toe	.95	1.64	2.65	.61	1.24	2.06
23. Epiphysis, proximal segment of 2d toe	.97	1.74	2.65	.63	1.19	2.05
24. Epiphysis of 3d metacarpal	.95	1.79	3.01	.65	1.13	1.94
25. Epiphysis, proximal segment of 5th finger	1.00	1.85	2.82	.65	1.19	2.07
26. Epiphysis, middle segment of 3d finger	1.01	1.97	3.31	.63	1.28	2.36
27. Epiphysis of 4th metacarpal	1.09	2.03	3.60	.75	1.29	2.17
28. EPiphysis, middle segment of 2d toe	.89	2.04	4.05	.49	1.18	2.24
29. Epiphysis, middle segment of 4th finger	1.00	2.05	3.24	.63	1.24	2.43
30. Epiphysis of 5th metacarpal	1.27	2.17	3.82	.86	1.37	2.35
31. First cuneiform of tarsus	.89	2.17	3.77	.50	1.43	2.82
32. Epiphysis of 1st metatarsal	1.39	2.18	3.12	.96	1.58	2.23
33. Epiphysis, middle segment of 2d finger	1.30	2.19	3.31	.67	1.36	2.54
34. Epiphysis, proximal segment of 1st toe	1.45	2.35	3.31	.89	1.55	2.47
35. Epiphysis, distal segment of 3d finger	1.31	2.41	3.72	.72	1.46	2.69
36. Triquetral of carpus	.49	2.43	5.47	.29	1.70	3.73
37. Epiphysis, distal segment of 4th finger	1.37	2.44	3.73	.73	1.52	2.82
38. Epiphysis, proximal segment of 5th toe	1.53	2.45	3.65	.97	1.73	2.67
39. Epiphysis of 1st metacarpal	1.45	2.59	4.32	.92	1.60	2.67
40. Second cuneiform of tarsus	1.19	2.65	4.21	.81	1.80	3.00
41. Epiphysis of 2d metatarsal	1.93	2.86	4.33	1.22	2.14	3.43
42. Greater trochanter of femur	1.92	2.96	4.35	.96	1.85	3.03
43. Epiphysis, proximal segment of 1st finger	1.84	3.00	4.57	.93	1.71	2.84
44. Navicular of tarsus	1.12	3.02	5.40	.77	1.94	3.58
45. Epiphysis, distal segment of 2d finger	1.80	3.17	4.97	1.06	2.50	3.29
46. Epiphysis, distal segment of 5th finger	2.06	3.29	4.98	1.01	1.96	3.45
47. Epiphysis, middle segment of 5th finger	1.94	3.40	5.84	.88	1.97	3.54
48. Proximal epiphysis of fibula	1.86	3.47	5.24	1.33	2.61	3.92
49. Epiphysis of 3d metatarsal	2.33	3.48	5.00	1.42	2.48	3.68
50. Epiphysis, distal segment of 5th toe	2.34	3.94	6.30	1.17	2.31	4.07
51. Patella of knee	2.55	4.00	5.96	1.47	2.48	4.01
52. Epiphysis of 4th metatarsal	2.92	4.02	5.74	1.77	2.84	4.05
53. Lunate of carpus	1.53	4.07	6.77	1.08	2.62	5.65
54. Epiphysis, distal segment of 3d toe	2.99	4.36	6.19	1.37	2.73	4.11
55. Epiphysis of 5th metatarsal	3.12	4.37	6.34	2.08	3.24	4.93
56. Epiphysis, distal segment of 4th toe	2.95	4.38	6.40	1.36	2.58	4.09

Table 1 (Continued)

	Percentiles					
	Boys			Girls		
Ossification Center	5th	50th	95th	5th	50th	95th
57. Epiphysis, distal segment of 2d toe	3.25	4.64	6.75	1.50	2.93	4.50
58. Capitulum of radius	3.00	5.21	7.97	2.26	3.87	6.28
59. Navicular of carpus	3.59	5.63	7.81	2.35	4.12	5.99
60. Greater multangular of carpus	3.53	5.87	8.97	1.94	4.08	6.36
61. Lesser multangular of carpus	3.12	6.22	8.50	2.38	4.17	6.01
62. Medial epicondyle of humerus	4.27	6.25	8.41	2.05	3.40	5.07
63. Distal epiphysis of ulna	5.25	7.10	9.07	3.29	5.37	7.63
64. Epiphysis of calcaneus	5.17	7.59	9.55	3.54	5.37	7.30
65. Olecranon of ulna	7.78	9.67	11.90	5.62	8.01	9.93
66. Lateral epicondyle of humerus	9.23	11.24	13.70	7.14	9.24	11.28
67. Tubercle of tibia	9.92	11.81	13.38	7.89	10.25	11.82
68. Adductor sesamoid of 1st finger	11.03	12.76	14.62	8.67	10.72	12.68
69. Os acetabulum of hip	11.90	13.54	15.32	9.60	11.47	13.39
70. Acromion of clavicle	12.15	13.74	15.48	10.32	11.92	13.79
71. Epiphysis, iliac crest of hip	12.03	14.03	15.91	10.81	12.79	15.31
72. Accessory epiphysis, coracoid process of scapula	12.74	14.35	16.31	10.37	12.21	14.37
73. Ischial tuberosity of hip	13.57	15.26	17.08	11.71	13.89	16.00

for a good functional result. Even so, the entire thickness of the growth cartilage has been breached, so that growth disturbance may occur. Fracture through the bony center of the epiphysis is more likely to result in growth disturbance than fracture through its unossified cartilage. In many instances, type III fracture is seen in older children in whom partial union of the shaft and epiphysis has already occurred. The fracture separates the ununited portion of the epiphysis from its united portion. as well as from its own contiguous metaphysis. In the distal tibia, the fracture may be obscured by the superimposed fibula.

In type IV fracture, the fracture line extends vertically through both the epiphysis and the adjacent shaft, traversing the growth cartilage. Accurate reduction is necessary, but even so the risk of growth disturbance is great. As in type III fractures, it is said to be less likely when the epiphyseal component of the fracture extends exclusively through unossified cartilage than when the fracture passes through the ossification center of the epiphysis.

Compression forces are responsible for type V fracture. The growth plate is crushed over a variable portion of its extent, and the damage leads to subsequent union of epiphysis and shaft. Radiographic diagnosis may be difficult; comparison with the opposite side is of great im-

portance, as is careful follow-up examination. It has been recommended that all epiphyseal injuries be followed for 6–12 months in order to identify growth disturbances.

Epiphyseal fractures may occur without involving the growth plate. These include avul-

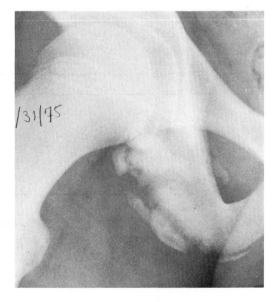

Fig. 6. Avulsion of the ischial apophysis with subsequent reaction in a 15-year-old boy. Too frequently these radiographic features are considered malignant when the appropriate history is not sought. (Courtesy of Dr. Stanford B. Rossiter, Redwood City, Calif.)

sion at the site of attachment of ligaments or periosteum, and displacement of an osteochondral fragment from the intraarticular margin of the epiphysis. These fractures do not cause growth disturbance, but the separated fragment may act as a foreign body.

Avulsion of an apophysis may occur without growth disturbance. Catterall[5] referred to apophyses as *traction epiphyses* that relate to muscle attachments. Characteristically the avulsion results from sudden muscle pull, usually in vigorous athletic activity. The anterior superior iliac spine may be avulsed by action of the sartorious muscle, the anterior inferior iliac spine by rectus femoris action, the lesser trochanter by the iliopsoas, and the ischial apophysis by the hamstrings (Fig. 6). Apophyseal avulsions occur most frequently in sprinters, football players, and jumpers.[10, 15]

The medial epicondyle of the humerus is avulsed by the action of throwing a ball, resulting in *Little-League elbow*. Avulsion of the cartilaginous spinous process of the tip of C-7 or T-1 has been likened to the adolescent equivalent of *clayshoveller's* disease in adults.[18]

THE BATTERED CHILD

The peculiar presentation of skeletal injury in abused children[3, 13] is generally a consequence of repetitive injury with exaggerated and prolonged repair. Similar features occur in comparable circumstances, such as congenital indifference to pain, organic sensory disturbance (eg, meningomyelocele), and unrecognized injury when immobilization is not employed. Even known injuries may present similar features if radiographed at an appropriate time after the trauma. The custom of obtaining follow-up films immediately after treatment and late (6 weeks) after cast removal to document bony union limits familiarity with the radiologic features of the intervening stages of healing.

The classic lesion in a battered child is a type I or type II epiphyseal separation. As noted previously, the cartilage-shaft junction is a site of relative weakness in skeletal structures and is particularly vulnerable to the shearing forces of combined torsion and tension, such as that exerted in sudden pulls on an extremity or shaking.[4] The critical diagnostic features are multiple injuries of this sort in different stages

of response and repair (Fig. 7A). These attest to repetitive injuries affecting multiple sites and interfering with healing. Hemorrhage is increased by repetition of injury, and consequently the amount and extent of callus formation are increased. When the callus calcifies sufficiently to become visible on radiographs, beginning in the third week after injury, exaggerated reparative changes are observed. Similarly, the replacement of bone damaged in later episodes exaggerates the postinjury "destruction." Because the original injury is unrecognized, forgotten, or denied, both destructive and productive aspects of bone repair following injury are prolonged by the microtrauma of motion superimposed on the original macrotrauma of epiphyseal separation. Some fractures may be well organized and obviously old, while others show active repair and destruction, and still others demonstrate only soft-tissue swelling in an area where the epiphyseal ossification center may or may not be malaligned with its subjacent shaft. Follow-up roentgenograms 2 to 3 weeks after the time of the first examination may demonstrate calcifying callus when the initial examination was nondiagnostic.

Diaphyseal fractures are seen, but a total skeletal survey is usually required to delimit the extent of injury, since skull fractures, rib fractures, vertebral fractures, and even fractures of the small bones of the hands have been described as manifestations of the battered child syndrome (Figs. 7B and C). A single fracture has diagnostic implications only if the history is inadequate to explain the nature of the fracture. Multiple fractures in varying stages of repair indicate multiple episodes of injury. They provide no information about the circumstances surrounding the injury, but they do provide a reason for investigation of these circumstances.

COMMENT

The general principles expressed above should help identify the common fractures in children and avoid overdiagnosis. This brief presentation cannot cover problems related to fractures of the jaw, skull, spine, pelvis, etc, but the same attention to detail in examination is applicable. To miss a minute fracture may not be as dangerous as to misdiagnose a fracture when it does not exist. The child tends to limit his own activity, and healing is usually prompt

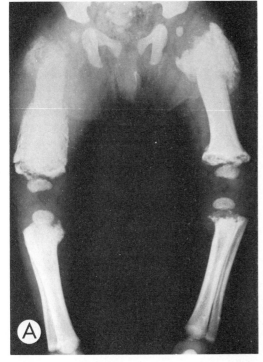

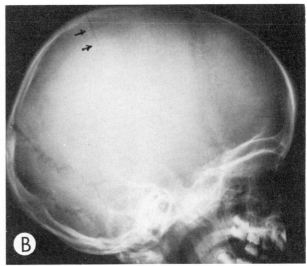

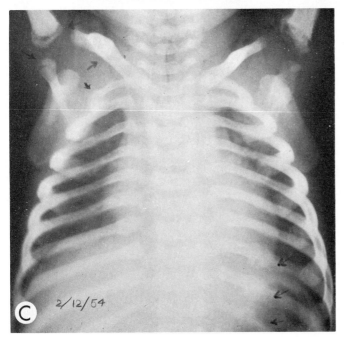

Fig. 7. Examples of bone lesions in the battered child: (A) Typical multiple metaphyseal fractures in different stages of repair. (Reproduced by permission from Silverman: Am J Roentgenol 69:413, 1953.) (B) A skull fracture like this discovered in a skeletal survey offers support for the diagnosis. The possibility of subdural hematoma must be considered, although they are more frequent without skull fracture.[4] (C) Healing fractures of ribs. These are more frequent in the battered child than obvious acute fractures. Same patient as in B. (Reproduced by permission from Silverman: Radiology 104:337–353, 1972.)

and complete. Unnecessary restriction of motion in a healthy child carries a greater hazard. The immobilization syndrome[7] is associated with hypercalcemia and its attendant complications; spontaneous premature union of epiphyses can occur from immobilization; vascular complications from tight-fitting casts or foreign bodies inserted in them by children have been described; emotional factors in restriction of activity in a child should not be overlooked. Attention to basic principles of radiologic diagnosis must be supplemented by an appreciation of the additional factors that apply specifically to infants and children.

REFERENCES

1. Blount WP: Fractures in Children (ed 1). Baltimore, Williams & Wilkins, 1955

2. Borden S: Roentgen recognition of acute plastic bowing of the forearm in children. Am J Roentgenol 125:524–530, 1975

3. Caffey JC: Some traumatic lesions in growing bones other than fractures and dislocations: Clinical and radiological features. The MacKenzie Davidson Memorial Lecture. Br J Radiol 30:225–238, 1957

4. Caffey J: On the theory and practice of shaking infants. Its potential residual effects of permanent brain damage and mental retardation. Am J Dis Child 124:161–169. 1972

5. Catterall A: Fractures in children, in Wilson JN (ed): Watson-Jones Fractures and Joint Injuries (ed 5). London, Churchill-Livingstone, 1976

6. Crowe JE, Swischuk IE: Acute bowing fractures of the forearm in children: A frequently missed injury. Am J Roentgenol 128:981–984, 1977

7. Dodd K, Graubarth H, Rapoport S: Hypercalcemia nephropathy and encephalopathy following immobilization; case report. Pediatrics 6:124–130, 1950

8. Garn SM, Rohmann CG, Silverman FN: Radiographic standards for postnatal ossification and tooth calcification. Med Radiogr Photogr 43:45–66, 1967

9. Griffiths AL: Fatigue fracture of the fibula in childhood. Arch Dis Child 27:552–557, 1952

10. Larson RL, McMahan RO: The epiphysis and the childhood athlete. JAMA 196:607–612, 1966

11. Rang M: Children's Fractures. Philadelphia, JB Lippincott, 1974

12. Salter RB, Harris WR: Injuries involving the epiphyseal plate. J Bone Joint Surg [Am] 45:587–622, 1963

13. Silverman FN: The roentgen manifestations of unrecognized skeletal trauma in infants. Am J Roentgenol 69:413–427, 1953; Unrecognized trauma in infants, the battered child syndrome and the syndrome of Ambroise Tardieu. Radiology 104:337–353, 1972

14. Swischuk LE: Spine and spinal cord trauma in the battered child syndrome. Radiology 92:733–738, 1969

15. Torg JS, Pollack H, Sweterlitsch P: The effect of competitive pitching on the shoulders and elbows of preadolescent baseball players. Pediatrics 49:267–272, 1972

16. Trueta J, Morgan JD: The vascular contribution to osteogenesis. I. Studies by the injection method. J Bone Joint Surg [Br] 42:97–109, 1960

17. Trueta J: The normal vascular anatomy of the human femoral head during growth. J Bone Joint Surg [Br] 39:358–394, 1957

18. Weston WJ: Clay shoveller's disease in adolescents (Schmitt's disease). Radiology 30:378–380, 1957

19. Wilkinson RH, Kirkpatrick JA Jr: Pediatric skeletal trauma. Curr Probl Diag Radiol 6:3–38, 1976

20. Wiot JF, Dorst JP: Less common fractures and dislocations of the wrist. Radiol Clin North Am 4:261–276, 1966

SUBJECT INDEX

SUBJECT INDEX

b
c
d
e
f
g
0 h
1 i
8 2 j